VALIDITY ASSESSMENT IN REHABILITATION

PSYCHOLOGY AND SETTINGS

ACADEMY OF REHABILITATION PSYCHOLOGY SERIES

Series Editors
Bruce Caplan, *Editor-in-Chief*
Timothy Elliott
Janet Farmer
Robert Frank
Barry Nierenberg
George Prigatano
Daniel Rohe
Stephen Wegener

Volumes in the Series

Ethics Field Guide: Applications in Rehabilitation Psychology
Thomas R. Kerkhoff and Stephanie L. Hanson

The Social Psychology of Disability
Dana Dunn

Disability-Affirmative Therapy: A Case Formulation Template for Clients with Disabilities
Rhoda Olkin

Validity Assessment in Rehabilitation Psychology and Settings
Dominic A. Carone and Shane S. Bush

Validity Assessment in Rehabilitation Psychology and Settings

Dominic A. Carone and Shane S. Bush

OXFORD
UNIVERSITY PRESS

OXFORD
UNIVERSITY PRESS

Oxford University Press is a department of the University of Oxford. It furthers
the University's objective of excellence in research, scholarship, and education
by publishing worldwide. Oxford is a registered trade mark of Oxford University
Press in the UK and certain other countries.

Published in the United States of America by Oxford University Press
198 Madison Avenue, New York, NY 10016, United States of America.

© Oxford University Press 2018

All rights reserved. No part of this publication may be reproduced, stored in
a retrieval system, or transmitted, in any form or by any means, without the
prior permission in writing of Oxford University Press, or as expressly permitted
by law, by license, or under terms agreed with the appropriate reproduction
rights organization. Inquiries concerning reproduction outside the scope of the
above should be sent to the Rights Department, Oxford University Press, at the
address above.

You must not circulate this work in any other form
and you must impose this same condition on any acquirer.

Library of Congress Cataloging-in-Publication Data
Names: Carone, Dominic A., author. | Bush, Shane S., 1965– author.
Title: Validity assessment in rehabilitation psychology and settings /
Dominic A. Carone and Shane S. Bush.
Description: New York, NY : Oxford University Press, [2018] |
Includes bibliographical references and index.
Identifiers: LCCN 2018006768 | ISBN 9780190674236
Subjects: LCSH: Rehabilitation—Psychological aspects. |
People with disabilities—Rehabilitation—Psychological aspects. |
Disability evaluation. | Psychiatric disability evaluation.
Classification: LCC RM930 .C37 2018 | DDC 617/.03—dc23
LC record available at https://lccn.loc.gov/2018006768

9 8 7 6 5 4 3 2 1

Printed by Webcom, Inc., Canada

This book is dedicated to the life and memory of our beloved friend and colleague, Dr. Manfred F. Greiffenstein (1952–2016), who helped revolutionize the field of validity assessment in clinical neuropsychology. His brilliant mind, quick wit, and insightful analysis will be missed by all. Most importantly, we will miss his friendship and collegiality.

Contents

1. Introduction: The Importance of Validity Assessment in Rehabilitation Psychology and Settings 1

2. Review of Performance Validity Assessment Methods 14

3. Review of Symptom Validity Assessment Methods 30

4. Validity Assessment in Patients with Brain Injury/Disease 42

5. Validity Assessment in Rehabilitation Patients without Brain Disorders 55

6. Lifespan Considerations in Validity Assessment 70

7. Interfacing with Rehabilitation Colleagues about Validity Assessment 85

8. Understanding and Managing Invalid Presentations in Rehabilitation Psychology and Settings 98

9. Forensic and Compensation-Seeking Applications of Validity Assessment in Rehabilitation Psychology and Settings 120

10. Ethical Considerations Involving Validity Assessment in Rehabilitation Psychology and Settings 128

REFERENCES 137
INDEX 159

1 Introduction
THE IMPORTANCE OF VALIDITY ASSESSMENT IN REHABILITATION PSYCHOLOGY AND SETTINGS

"REHABILITATION" COMES FROM the Latin word "rehabilitare," meaning "to make fit." As such, the overarching goal of all rehabilitation professionals should be to help patients make improvements in their ability to function following disease, illness, or injury. Unfortunately, there are various factors that interfere with implementation of this goal such that patients indefinitely remain in the status quo or get worse over time. These factors include but are not limited to medical complications (e.g., chronic pain, pressure ulcers, deep vein thromboses), socioeconomic problems (e.g., low educational attainment, poor social support, inadequate insurance), mental health problems (e.g., major depressive disorder, personality disorders, agitation), iatrogenesis (negative outcomes caused by a healthcare provider), and poor compliance with treatment and assessments (e.g., poor effort on performance-based tests, refusal to participate in therapy, leaving against medical advice, frequent no-shows and cancellations, and overreporting or underreporting of symptoms). In many instances, several of these factors are intertwined in the same patient, resulting in a complex multifactorial clinical picture.

The purpose of this book is to focus predominantly on one of these factors (i.e., invalid responding due to poor effort, overreporting, and underreporting) and to explain why it is of critical importance to understand and assess these issues in rehabilitation settings. In so doing, chapters are provided on the assessment of performance and symptom validity (chapters 2 and 3) in diverse populations (chapters 4, 5, and 6). Practical clinical information is also provided regarding interdisciplinary communication of symptom and performance validity issues (chapter 7), how to understand and manage invalid presentations (chapter 8), applications of symptom and performance validity assessment to forensic and compensation-seeking contexts (chapter 9), and ethical considerations of symptom and performance validity assessment (chapter 10). This book is primarily intended for rehabilitation professionals who are new to the topic of symptom and performance validity assessment who seek a greater understanding of the topic to assist with their clinical work. However, we also believe that the content of this book will be of interest to those experienced in this area (e.g., clinical neuropsychologists), particularly those who work in rehabilitation settings.

Validity, Symptom Validity, and Performance Validity

Validity, in its broadest sense, refers to how logically sound and well founded something is. In science, validity refers to the extent that a concept, conclusion, or measurement is well founded and accurately corresponds to reality. In psychological assessment, "validity" is typically used to refer to "the degree to which evidence and theory support the interpretation of test scores for proposed use" (American Educational Research Association, 2014, p. 11). During training, psychologists learn about four main types of validity with regard to psychological testing: (1) face validity (the extent to which a test *appears* to measure a certain criterion at face value, although it is technically not a true form of validity but actually a measure of social acceptability), (2) construct validity (the extent to which a test measures the construct that it claims to measure), (3) content validity (the extent to which a test measures the various content associated with the intended construct), and (4) criterion validity (the extent to which test performance is related to an outcome) (Kaplan & Saccuzzo, 2013). Within these broad constructs of test validity are various subtypes of validity. One example is predictive validity, which is a type of criterion validity that measures the extent that test performance predicts scores on some criterion measure. Psychologists consider these various aspects of test validity (and reliability) when selecting assessment instruments for use in clinical practice in a manner consistent with the ethics code of the American Psychological Association (2010).

In contrast to test validity, symptom and performance validity focus on the validity of the patient's responses and behaviors. Although ways to assess for positive and/or negative impression management on personality tests have long been covered in graduate textbooks on psychological assessment (Anastasi & Urbina, 1997; Cohen, Swerdlik, & Smith, 1992; Kaplan & Saccuzzo, 2013), performance validity was not a topic that was traditionally covered. Modern collegiate textbooks sometimes contain no information on symptom and performance validity (Gregory, 2014) or sometimes just provide brief reference (Hogan, 2015) that pales in comparison to coverage of test validity.

The current version of the *Standards for Educational and Psychological Testing* (American Educational Research Association, 2014) does not contain an explicit specific standard mentioning the need to assess for symptom and performance validity but it does contain some related information on the topic. For example, standard 1.10 states, "attention should be drawn to any features of validation data collection that are likely to differ from typical operational testing conditions and that could plausibly influence test performances" (p. 26). One such condition mentioned is test-taker motivation, but the context is limited to validation data collection. The background section on reliability mentions that a number of factors could significantly affect reliability/precision, which can lead to significant misinterpretations of test results if not taken into account, but does not specifically mention motivation. Standard 6.6 states, "Reasonable efforts should be made to ensure the integrity of test scores by eliminating opportunities for test takers to attain scores by fraudulent or deceptive means" (p. 116). However, the context of this standard is about preventing people from cheating to do well, and there is discussion of using modern technology (e.g., computer analysis of erasure patterns) to detect such cheating. Of most relevance to the topic of this book, standard 9.13 states, "a test taker's scores should not be interpreted in isolation; other relevant information that may lead to alternative explanations for the examinee's test performance should be considered" (p. 145) and mentions low motivation as the first obvious explanation for low scores. Last, although not a standard, the chapter on psychological testing and assessment mentions that in instances involving legal issues it is important to assess response bias such as exaggeration of cognitive and emotional symptoms to maximize financial gain. It is further stated, "In forming an assessment opinion, it is necessary to interpret the test scores with informed knowledge relating to the available validity and reliability evidence" (p. 162).

Although books about neuropsychological assessment (Lezak, Howieson, Bigler, & Tranel, 2012; Morgan & Ricker, 2008; Strauss, Sherman, & Spreen, 2006) contain detailed information about symptom and performance validity assessment, the topic is not covered at all in *The Oxford Handbook of Rehabilitation Psychology* (Kennedy, 2012). Symptom validity assessment and malingering is covered in the second edition of the *APA Handbook of Rehabilitation Psychology* (Frank, Rosenthal, & Caplan, 2010), but only in the context of a chapter on forensic psychological evaluations, and is absent from the clinically oriented chapter on neuropsychological practice in rehabilitation. In the forthcoming third edition of the *APA Handbook of Rehabilitation Psychology*, Bush and Rush (in press) devote considerable coverage to validity assessment under the broader topic of psychological assessment in rehabilitation contexts. Bush and Rush (in press) state, "The results of psychological assessment are only meaningful if the psychologist has confidence that the patient responded honestly to questions and put forth good effort on cognitive and sensorimotor tests." In the most recent edition of the mammoth, 1,232-page *Braddom's Physical Medicine and Rehabilitation* (Cifu, 2016), there is only one broad paragraph about symptom and performance validity assessment (which is limited to neuropsychological evaluations) and five mentions throughout the book of malingering as possible explanations for patient presentations. Malingering, which is the intentional production of false or grossly exaggerated physical or psychological symptoms motivated by external incentives (American Psychiatric Association, 2013), is just one possible reason why a patient may respond in an invalid manner. Because of the limited coverage that symptom and performance validity assessment receives in general psychological assessment training and rehabilitation context, we chose to focus the current book on this topic.

For those who are new to the topic of symptom and performance validity assessment, the terminology can be confusing because it has evolved over time. The term "symptom validity testing" (SVT) was originally used by Pankratz (1979) to describe a two-alternative forced-choice procedure to identify functional sensory deficits. Even though the test required the patient to perform a function (e.g., guessing whether the stimulus was present or not), the term "symptom validity" was used because the technique was measuring the validity of a patient's reported symptom (e.g., sensory loss) during an interview. Pankratz (1983) later used the technique to assess feigned memory deficits, and the term "SVT" continued to be used in the literature. By the mid-1990s, numerous freestanding and embedded SVTs were developed (see chapter 2). Freestanding SVTs are those created for the express purpose of assessing valid responses, whereas embedded SVTs are those that are extracted from tests not originally designed for that purpose.

Over time, confusion began to emerge about why SVTs were named as such when there were self-report scales that existed to assess the validity of self-reported symptoms. The best-known examples are the validity scales from the Minnesota Multiphasic Personality Inventory-2 (MMPI-2) (Butcher, Dahlstrom, Graham, Tellegen, & Kaemmer, 1989). Additional confusion was caused by the seemingly interchangeable use of the term "SVT" with terms such as "effort tests," "tests of response bias," and "malingering tests." To address the problem with terminology,

Larrabee (2012) proposed that the term "SVT" be used to refer to a test that evaluates the validity of a patient's responses on self-report scales and that the term "performance validity test" or "PVT" be used to refer to a test that evaluated the validity of a patient's responses on performance-based tests. He also suggested that these terms replace less descriptive terms such as tests of "effort" and "response bias." This new proposal was met with widespread acceptance and has become the way that these terms are currently used.

In addition to responses to test items and effort on tests, the accuracy of patient responses during clinical interviews needs to be considered. For example, research has demonstrated that persons with a history of traumatic brain injury who are undergoing litigation tend in inflate their scholastic achievement (Greiffenstein, Baker, & Johnson-Greene, 2002). In the context of assessment of rehabilitation patients, Bush and Rush (in press) stated, "Accurate case conceptualizations depend on patients providing accurate responses to interview questions about their background, including education level, work history, substance use history, history of a learning disability, history of a psychiatric disorder, and so forth." Bush (2014) proposed using the term "response validity" to describe self-reported information, which can intentionally or unintentionally be incorrect, incomplete, or otherwise misleading.

Hartman (2002) noted that a freestanding psychological validity tests should meet eight criteria. First, the test should measure the concept it was designed to assess (willingness to exert a basic effort) and be insensitive to cognitive dysfunction. In other words, the test should have adequate sensitivity and specificity (see chapter 2). The first criterion would better be stated as the test being *relatively* insensitive to cognitive impairment, because no effort test could technically be completely insensitive to the most extreme forms of cognitive impairment. Second, the test should appear to the patient to be an assessment of cognition as opposed to effort. Third, the test should measure abilities likely to be exaggerated by patients claiming brain damage. Fourth, the test should have strong norms underlying the test results such that it can withstand scientific scrutiny and meet legal criteria for admissible evidence in court. Fifth, validation studies should involve healthy controls, patient populations, and individuals who are suspected and/or verified malingerers in forensic or disability assessment conditions. Sixth, the test should be difficult to fake or coach. Seventh, the test should be relatively easy to administer. Eighth, the test should be supported by continuing research. Not all validity tests discussed in this book meet all of these criteria, but these are excellent guidelines for test users to consider when determining which test to use or whether a test used by another healthcare provider was adequate for the specific clinical situation.

Why Assess Symptom and Performance Validity?

Any healthcare provider collecting patient data should want to know whether the data is valid because it is relied on to make diagnostic decisions, inferences about level of functioning, treatment decisions, and other recommendations. If the obtained information is not valid, misdiagnosis, misstatements, improper treatment, and improper recommendations can result, which can all result in significant harm to the patient. This is not a topic that is unique to neuropsychology and rehabilitation professions. For example, when radiologists discovered that patient breathing motion artifact was the most common cause of misdiagnosed pulmonary embolisms on pulmonary computerized tomography angiography (CTA) studies, they recommended improvements in the quality of the examinations and increased awareness in the profession about this diagnostic pitfall (Hutchinson, Navin, Marom, Truong, & Bruzzi, 2015). Pulmonologists developed methods to determine whether forced vital capacity (a measure of forceful breathing effort) measures are valid based on the amount of effort the patient exerts (Al-Ashkar, Mehra, & Mazzone, 2003). Those authors specifically noted, "Results that were not reproducible may not accurately reflect the patient's true lung pathology" (p. 877). As another example, recognizing that some patients simulate ophthalmologic diseases or disorders, Incesu (2013) recommended increased awareness in the profession about this problem and the use of several simulation examination techniques during ophthalmological examinations. In each of these examples, healthcare providers from diverse professions recognized the importance of validity assessment, raised awareness about the topic to their colleagues, and promoted improvements or techniques to improve the quality of the examination process.

As noted earlier, in the rehabilitation profession, invalid responding is a factor that can interfere with rehabilitation goals and can lead to patients failing to improve or worsening over time. Recent research has shown that patients who show inadequate effort on cognitive evaluations have more healthcare use (e.g., more Emergency Department and inpatient visits) compared to patients who exert adequate effort (Horner, VanKirk, Dismuke, Turner, & Muzzy, 2014). If such findings extend to outpatient rehabilitation settings (which is reasonable to suspect), then increased service use by patients exerting inadequate effort will yield more billing charges and outpatient revenue but will also interfere with appointment availability for other patients and runs the risk of overstraining healthcare resources.

As noted in *Braddom's Physical Medicine and Rehabilitation* (Cifu, 2016), there is potential for rehabilitation patients to be involved in litigation, which increases the chances of exaggerated cognitive and physical presentations and can place the rehabilitation professional in dual roles (e.g., expert witness or fact witness/treating clinician). This is a concern not only for psychologists and physicians but also for other rehabilitation professionals. For example, in the first study using objective tests of cognitive effort in occupational therapy (OT) practice, Fleming and Rucas (2015) found that 48% of consecutive patients evaluated in an outpatient medical-legal context failed one or two effort tests. This led the authors to propose the following standard for occupational therapists: "When there are cognitive and/or psychosocial complaints OR there is a question about cognitive functioning, we should first ensure the validity of our assessment findings and only then draw conclusions from our formal assessment results" (p. 7).

In a survey of board certified neuropsychologists, a high base rate (i.e., 41%) of symptom exaggeration or probable malingering was found in patients with a history of mild traumatic brain injury (Mittenberg, Patton, Canyock, & Condit, 2002) who were litigating or compensation seeking. This is particularly relevant to outpatient rehabilitation settings, given the veritable explosion of concussion clinics across the United States. The same study also revealed that the base rate for symptom exaggeration or probable malingering was high (39%) in patients with fibromyalgia or chronic fatigue but low (between 2% and 9%) in litigating or compensation-seeking patients with vascular dementia, moderate or severe traumatic brain injury, and seizure disorders. Thus, the survey results show that symptom exaggeration and malingering is reported to be more likely in patients with no (or fewer) objective biomarkers of neurological injury or disease (e.g., neuroimagining or neurophysiological findings) and vice versa. This violation of dose-response relationships (i.e., worse function despite less documented disease) has been found on tests of motor function (Greiffenstein, Baker, & Gola, 1996), performance validity tests (Haber & Fichtenberg, 2006; Heinly, Greve, Bianchini, Love, & Brennan, 2005), symptom validity tests (Miller & Donders, 2001; Youngjohn, Wershba, Stevenson, Sturgeon, & Thomas, 2011), and clinical rehabilitation settings (Carone, 2008; Sherer et al., 2015).

Although symptom and performance validity assessment is important in medicolegal contexts, it is also important in other contexts such as research settings and clinical work. For example, poor effort has been documented among volunteer research participants to range from to 2% to 56% (An, Zakzanis, & Joordens, 2012; DeRight & Jorgensen, 2015; Ross et al., 2016; Silk-Eglit et al., 2014). Although some evaluations are clearly identified as medicolegal from the outset, many clinical cases (i.e., referred by healthcare providers) occur in the context of compensation seeking (e.g., a disability application, lawsuit, workers' compensation claim). In clinical settings, factors that can contribute to invalid data besides medicolegal proceedings include (1) avoidance of responsibilities (e.g., work, school, military service), (2) attempts to convince a healthcare provider about the significance of one's symptoms, (3) attention seeking (e.g., factitious disorder), (4) appearing to fall asleep at times during testing, (5) attempts to obtain medications (e.g., narcotics), (6) personality and emotional variables (e.g., sense of entitlement, neediness, anger, personality disorders), (7) somatization, (8) reinforced behavior patterns (e.g., in chronic pain), (9) cognitive distortions (e.g., depressive negativistic thinking, misattribution bias), (10) iatrogenesis, (11) opposition to the evaluation, and (12) poor insight and denial (for those underreporting symptoms) (Carone, Iverson, & Bush, 2010). Thus, validity assessment is an important issue that goes well beyond the assessment of malingering.

Who Should Assess Performance and Symptom Validity?

There has been no other discipline that has done more to advance the science of symptom and performance validity assessment than clinical neuropsychology. This is exemplified by the veritable explosion of SVTs and PVTs published by clinical neuropsychologists since the 1990s (see chapters 2 and 3). Clinical neuropsychology has also been at the forefront of promoting the need for the widespread use of symptom and performance validity assessment. This is demonstrated by the position papers and consensus statements the National Academy of Neuropsychology (NAN) (Bush et al., 2005) and the American Academy of Clinical Neuropsychology (AACN, 2007; Chafetz et al., 2015; Heilbronner, Sweet, Morgan, Larrabee, & Millis, 2009) emphasizing the need to assess symptom and performance validity in all, or nearly all, evaluations. The NAN position paper was significant because it was the first time that any national organization of healthcare professionals expressly endorsed the routine use of symptom and performance validity assessment in forensic and clinical contexts. Because of the unique role clinical neuropsychology has played in promoting and developing the science of symptom and performance validity assessment, clinical neuropsychologists have the most expertise in performing these types of assessments.

An important question is whether symptom and performance validity assessment in psychological evaluations should be limited only to clinical neuropsychologists. We are mindful that some will hold the position that the answer to this question is yes. However, we do not believe this is a tenable position for several reasons. First, in some rehabilitation settings there are no neuropsychologists available or not enough neuropsychologists available to serve the patient volume. Second, in these situations, it is not uncommon for rehabilitation psychologists to perform cognitive testing, and it is within the scope of practice of rehabilitation psychologists to do so (Hibbard & Cox, 2010; Stiers et al., 2015). Third, many rehabilitation psychologists have some form of education and training in clinical neuropsychology even though it usually does not meet aspirational neuropsychology training standards (National Academy of Neuropsychology, 1998; Sweet, Perry, Ruff, Shear, & Guidotti Breting, 2012). Thus, although both professions have unique skills and competencies that are not interchangeable, there is some degree of overlap between the two professions (in both directions). This overlap can lead to territorial friction, which may or not be warranted depending on the specific situation, the educational and training backgrounds of the individuals involved, and the team dynamics.

While recognizing that this interdisciplinary tension sometimes exists, we know of no set of guidelines or consensus statement that limits symptom and performance validity assessment to clinical neuropsychologists. In fact, the most recent position paper published on validity assessment by the AACN (Chafetz et al., 2015) states in the recommendation section for the use of SVTs and PVTs in consultative evaluations for the Social Security Administration (SSA) that *"All psychologist consultants and psychological examiners (PEs)* working within the SSA disability program should be provided with specific training on how PVTs and SVTs can be used to enhance disability determination decisions" (p. 14, emphasis added). The more general term "psychologist" was used in that article seven times, whereas the term "neuropsychologist" was only used once, likely due to recognition that neuropsychologists are not the only type of psychologist performing such evaluations. Use of the more general term "psychologist" makes sense, especially when considering that all clinical psychologists learn early in graduate education that determining the validity of test results is the first step in the interpretation of omnibus personality tests such as the MMPI-2. Limiting rehabilitation psychologists to the assessment of symptom validity on personality tests but not performance validity on cognitive tests does not make sense, because the examiner, referral source, and others need to know whether the results are valid in both situations. This view is supported by position papers from other psychological organizations (British Psychological Society, 2009; Bush, Heilbronner, & Ruff, 2014).

Despite the situation just described, it has been our experience is that it is rare for rehabilitation psychologists to assess for symptom and performance validity beyond the automatic calculation of validity scales on omnibus personality tests. The main reasons for this appear to be: (1) the topic is not discussed much among rehabilitation psychologists compared to clinical neuropsychologist (see Table 1.1 for an example); (2) a tendency in the rehabilitation community to take patient reporting and performance at face value; (3) a bias toward *perceived* patient advocacy responsibilities versus the need for objectivity, accuracy, and honesty (Carone, 2015); (4) an incorrect belief that behavioral observations and clinical judgment alone are sufficient ground to make validity determinations (see Guilmette, 2013, for a critique of this approach); (5) a perception that validity assessment is a

TABLE 1.1

PubMed: Title and Abstract Hits for Combinations of Search Terms

	Neuropsychological	Rehabilitation psychology	Neuropsychology	Rehabilitation psychologists	Neuropsychologists
Effort	512	1*	79	0	24
Malingering	272	0	61	0	32
Symptom validity	164	0	40	0	13
Performance validity	89	0	35	0	6
Response bias	85	0	13	0	8
Invalid	80	0	19	0	4
Validity testing	72	0	25	0	12
Poor effort	53	0	3	0	3
Exaggeration	49	0	8	0	8
Effort testing	30	0	6	0	2
Feigning	18	0	4	0	3
Fake bad	7	0	2	0	1

Note: Search terms were separated by the word "AND" for combined results. Only title and abstract searches were performed, to better isolate the focus of returned studies. Journal titles were not used in the searches to prevent misleading results because neuropsychological studies are sometimes published in rehabilitation journals. The term "neurorehabilitation" was not used, because that term encompasses other professions besides rehabilitation psychology (including neuropsychology). Search terms in each table row were listed in descending order based on the number of hits when combined with the search term "neuropsychological." An example of the way the search terms were typed in the search field is as follows: (neuropsychology['Title/Abstract']) AND validity testing['Title/Abstract'].

Searches were performed on September 9, 2016.

Source: http://www.ncbi.nlm.nih.gov/sites/entrez

*The one returned hit for the combination of "effort" and "rehabilitation psychology" was for an article (Diller, 2005) that refers to "the effort to reach people to overcome or adapt to limitations." Thus, the returned article is not related to validity assessment. Reference: Diller, L. (2005). Pushing the frames of reference in traumatic brain injury rehabilitation. *Archives of Physical Medicine and Rehabilitation, 86*, 1075–1080.

neuropsychology-only technique; (6) an incorrect belief that validity only needs to be assessed in litigating patients; (7) social discomfort in discussing failed validity results with patients, family members, and other healthcare providers; (8) not wanting to risk patient complaints/reprisals; (9) a belief that healthcare providers should not be "detectives"; and (10) fear of false positive classification (i.e., classifying data as invalid when it is not).

At the time of this book's publication, with the exception of clinical neuropsychology, we are not aware of any mainstream national organization of healthcare professionals (e.g., American Board of Rehabilitation Psychology, American Board of Physical Medicine and Rehabilitation, American Medical Association; American College of Environmental and Occupational Medicine, American Occupational Therapy Association, American Physical Therapy Association) that has endorsed the routine use of symptom and performance validity assessment in clinical evaluations, and this continues to be a problem. Without the sanctioned and recommended use of validity assessment by such organizations, non-neuropsychology healthcare providers may sometimes encounter resistance when trying to conduct and/or publish scientific studies about this topic. For example, Fleming and Rucas (personal communication, September 13, 2016) published their research in a neuropsychology journal after it was rejected from two OT journals. In addition, despite the call for an OT-specific PVT proposed by Fleming and Rucas (2015), formal scientific explorations of performance validity assessment as a proposed standard of practice within OT have been discouraged to date, with no further publications on the topic at the time this book went to publication. Per Reema Shafi (personal communication, September 13, 2016), an occupational therapist in Canada, when her research grant application on performance validity assessment stated that it was "imperative for OT clinicians to substantiate client complaints, void of any biases, before determining needs," a grant reviewer stated that this was indicative of an alliance with the insurance industry even though such an alliance was reportedly not present. In addition, opportunities to present on the topic to peers in an effort to mobilize and disseminate the existing body of knowledge have reportedly been declined without any explanation (R. Shafi, personal communication, September 13, 2016).

Our main impetus for writing this book is to raise awareness of the importance of assessing symptom and performance validity in rehabilitation settings and the need for validity assessment to become common practice for all rehabilitation professions just as it has in clinical neuropsychology for children and adolescents (Brooks, Ploetz, & Kirkwood, 2016) and adults (Martin, Schroeder, & Odland, 2015). The interested reader is referred to these studies for tables of commonly used PVTs and SVTs.

Rehabilitation professionals should of course have a good working knowledge of the topic of symptom and performance validity assessment and a detailed understanding of any SVT or PVT intended for use in clinical practice. Clinicians must avoid warning patients about the purpose of these instruments, avoid coaching, and be prepared to report the results accurately in the report and during feedback sessions. While this book does not purport to equip rehabilitation professionals with the requisite working knowledge to assess symptom and performance validity, we believe that it provides an important introduction and educational framework for the profession to more proactively address this topic. Rehabilitation professionals who are interested in learning more about this topic should familiarize themselves with the NAN and AACN consensus statements and position papers, read peer-reviewed scientific literature on the topic, attend professional workshops on validity assessment, join or create professional listservs where these topics are regularly discussed, and seek additional training and consultation with neuropsychology colleagues who are familiar with these assessment methods. While we have our own preferred validity assessment measures, we feel it is best for clinicians to use the information in this book and elsewhere to decide what assessment measures they would like to use.

Lastly, it cannot be automatically assumed that nonpsychologist rehabilitation professionals can use existing psychological validity tests without permission from the test publisher due to established user qualification standards that require a high level of expertise in test interpretation. In some instances, the same test publisher will have different user standards depending on the sophistication of the test and required background knowledge and training in psychological assessment, statistics, and ethics. For example, the publisher of the Word Memory Test (Green, 2003) has only made the test available to licensed psychologists, whereas all other validity tests published by the company can be purchased by licensed psychologists and physicians. In fact, one commonly used PVT, the Medical Symptom Validity Test (MSVT) (Green 2004a) was originally developed in response to the demand by some physicians for an efficient cognitive effort measure (Carone, 2009). However, other healthcare professionals (e.g., speech therapists, physical therapists, occupational therapists) are prohibited by the test publisher from purchasing and using these tests with rare exceptions, such as two occupational therapists (Fleming & Rucas, 2015) who were permitted to use the MSVT with psychologist supervision. With regard to self-report-based questionnaires developed by psychologists to assess the validity of reported symptoms (e.g., pain, memory problems), permitted use of these tests by nonpsychologists and nonphysicians will depend on the qualification standards established by the test publisher/author and the sophistication of the test (e.g., brief checklists versus omnibus tests of personality with hundreds of test items and extensive clinical scales that require advanced training in psychological assessment to interpret). Ultimately, as Carone (2013) previously noted, it is important for nonpsychologist healthcare providers to develop profession-specific validity tests (or better validity tests) in their specific profession. This is partly because there are functions (e.g., speech articulation, balance, ocular motility) commonly assessed by members of nonpsychology professions that will not be adequately covered by psychological validity assessment measures. Development of profession-specific validity tests would also eliminate questions of test user qualifications when used by members of that specific profession.

Summary and Conclusions

It is critical for healthcare providers to establish the validity of patient data before relying on it to make diagnostic decisions, inferences about a patient's level of function, treatment decisions, and other recommendations. Symptom and performance validity assessment is an essential component of neuropsychological evaluations but is currently vastly underutilized among rehabilitation psychologists and other rehabilitation professionals. We believe that this is a topic that deserves much greater attention by the rehabilitation psychology community, other rehabilitation professions, and any other healthcare professionals using psychological or cognitive tests. Lastly, we propose that the next version of the *Standards for Educational Testing and Psychological Testing* (2014) include a specific standard on the importance of assessing symptom and performance validity in diverse settings (e.g., clinical, forensic, research).

2   Review of Performance Validity Assessment Methods

THE GOAL OF this chapter is to provide the rehabilitation professional new to validity assessment with a general overview of performance validity tests (PVTs), examples of some commonly used PVTs along with supportive research, and some important issues surrounding the use and interpretation of PVTs. We did not aim to provide a detailed accounting of the many different types of PVTs available for use with adults and children, as we have provided this information elsewhere (Bush & Bass, 2015; Carone, 2015a; Carone & Bush, 2013; Deright & Carone, 2015) as have others (Bianchini, Mathias, & Greve, 2001; Boone, 2007; Iverson, 2007; Kirkwood, 2015; Larrabee, 2005; Lynch, 2004; Reynolds & Horton, 2012). The interested reader is referred to those writings for more detailed information.

Terminology

As noted in the introduction, a "performance validity test" or "PVT" refers to a test that is used to infer the validity of performance on tests of cognitive and sensory-motor ability. There are two types of PVTs that use scores—freestanding and embedded. Freestanding PVTs are those that were originally designed for the express purpose of assessing performance validity. Embedded PVTs are those that are extracted from tests (i.e., ability measures) not originally designed for the purpose of validity assessment. In addition to these types of PVTs, there are also qualitative measures of validity assessment that use behavioral observations (see later section in this chapter for a review) as opposed to scores to determine whether a patient's behavioral presentation appears valid.

Finding the Right Balance: Sensitivity, Specificity, and Predictive Values

Performance validity tests provide information on whether a patient puts forth adequate effort to do well. For PVTs to work as intended, they need to have the highest possible specificity rate (i.e., at least 90%) such that they correctly classify performance as valid when it actually is valid while *simultaneously* having a high sensitivity rate such that they correctly classify invalid performance when it is actually invalid (Schroeder, Twumasi-Ankrah, Baade, & Marshall, 2012). In other words, it is very important for PVTs to have a high true negative rate (specificity) and a high true positive rate (sensitivity). Technically, sensitivity is calculated by taking the total number of true positives and dividing it by the total number of people with the condition of interest (true positives and false negatives). Specificity is calculated by taking the total number of true negatives and dividing it by the total number of people without the condition of interest (true negatives and false positives). Clinicians need to avoid both type I errors (i.e., determining that valid effort is invalid) and type II errors (determining that invalid effort is valid). In less statistical language, clinicians need to be accurate with their determinations regarding effort.

There is typically an inverse relationship between specificity and sensitivity such that one typically falls as the other rises. Thus, tests with higher specificity typically have lower sensitivity and vice versa. Test developers set empirical cutoffs on freestanding and embedded PVTs that are primarily designed to maximize specificity (at the cost of lower sensitivity) because it is considered more important to avoid false positive classifications (classifying performance as invalid when it is actually valid) than to avoid false negative classifications (classifying performance as valid when it is actually invalid). For example, it would be worse to suggest that someone is malingering when he or she is not than to fail to identify malingering when it occurs. Reduction of false positives is further enhanced by using multiple methods to assess validity. Developers of freestanding PVTs attempt to achieve a balance between sensitivity and specificity by designing tests that *appear* to be challenging measures of ability that are actually very easy tasks that require minimal ability. Hence, motivation to do well on such tests is generally all that is required to obtain a passing score even in individuals with severe neurological conditions (e.g., severe traumatic brain injury [TBI]). Developers of embedded PVTs typically set such cutoffs by presenting sensitivity and specificity rates regarding task performance of patients independently classified as probably or definitely malingering versus a patient group with no identified incentive to perform poorly and/or health controls. For some measures, test publishers or other researchers provide such psychometric information for various known groups (e.g., patients with various disorders) so that clinicians can choose a cutoff score that seems most appropriate for a given population. For more detailed information on setting empirical cutoffs for PVTs, the interested reader is referred to Greve and Bianchini (2004).

Related statistical information that is important to understand in the PVT literature is positive predictive value (PPV) and negative predictive value (NPV), which are also known as positive and negative predictive power, respectively. Positive predictive value is the probability that someone truly has the condition of interest when a positive test result is obtained. This is determined by taking the number of true positives and dividing it by the sum of true positives and false positives. As an analogy to a medical test, if it is known that people without breast cancer rarely have a positive test result on a certain breast cancer screening test, then one can be very confident that a person has breast cancer if a positive test result is obtained. Negative predictive value is the probability that someone does not have the condition of interest when a negative result is obtained. This is determined by taking the number of true negatives and dividing it by the sum of true negatives and false negatives. As another analogy, if it is known that a breast cancer screening test rarely misses people with breast cancer, then one can be very confident that a person does not have breast cancer if a negative breast cancer screening result is obtained. In this way, PPV and NPV are dependent on the prevalence of the condition in the sample being tested whereas sensitivity and specificity rates are characteristics of the test.

Performance Validity Test Paradigms

Most freestanding PVTs are based on a memory paradigm because poor memory is a very common type of cognitive complaint (if not the most common) of patients presenting for a neuropsychological assessments. Many other types of cognitive complaints are also potentially associated in some way with memory such as problems with word finding, multitasking, and attention and concentration. For example, a patient may report "forgetting" a person's name, "forgetting" what to do next when moving from one task to another, or "forgetting" what to do when distracted. The association of forgetfulness with other cognitive functions likely further increases the sensitivity of PVTs that use a memory paradigm. Other cognitive complaints (e.g., visual-constructional problems, slowed processing speed, and speech dysfluency) and sensory-motor complaints have less ostensible associations with memory problems, and there are other PVTs that exist to evaluate validity within these domains, mostly of the embedded variety (for a detailed review, see Victor, Boone, & Kulick, 2013; Victor, Kulick, & Boone, 2013).

The vast majority of freestanding PVTs use a forced choice paradigm in which the patient is required to choose between one of two responses to provide the correct answer. One advantage of this approach is that performance that is below chance at a statistically significant level provides strong evidence of intentionally biased responding. The reason for this is because even if the patient had never been exposed to the test stimuli previously, he or she would be expected to get approximately 50% correct by chance. A disadvantage of forced choice PVTs is that they are readily identifiable to patients who have been warned/coached about the use of such tests. For this reason, a multimethod approach to validity assessment is recommended (Bush et al., 2005). Multimethod approaches use methods beyond testing to evaluate validity such as qualitative behavioral observations (Carone, 2015b) but also use PVTs in non-forced-choice formats. By definition, non-forced-choice PVTs allow for a range of responses and work by evaluating patterns of unrealistically slow responses, errors, and patterns of responses when compared to performance of patients with neurological conditions who are not being evaluated in a compensation-seeking context. Because most PVTs were developed within the context of TBI assessment, many of the examples of PVTs in this chapter include some mention of TBI. However, we emphasized several studies that were performed in rehabilitation settings. Performance validity test use with patients who have a history of TBI and non-TBI are a specific focus of chapters 3 and 4, respectively.

FORCED CHOICE FREESTANDING PERFORMANCE VALIDITY TESTS

The Medical Symptom Validity Test (MSVT) (Green, 2004) and the Word Memory Test (WMT) (Green, 2003) are two related tests that are among the top three PVTs used in neuropsychological assessments (Martin, Schroeder, & Odland, 2015). Both tests involve the computerized presentations of word pairs that have very strong semantic associations (e.g., hot cold). An oral version of the WMT is available, which can be helpful in situations (e.g., inpatient rehabilitation units) where computer/laptop access may be difficult (Hoskins, Binder, Chaytor, Williamson, & Drane, 2010). The MSVT has 10 word pairs and the WMT has 20 word pairs. By using a high volume of words, these tests appear to patients to be a genuine test of memory ability. In fact, there are more words on the MSVT and WMT than on commonly used measures of verbal learning and ability. However, unlike actual tests of verbal learning and memory, the very strong semantic associations between the MSVT and WMT word pairs generally make them extremely easy to learn, even to most individuals with severe neurological conditions. After the word pairs are presented two consecutive times, the patient is immediately presented with a forced choice Immediate Recognition (IR) subtest, in which one word from the list is presented along with a foil (e.g., hot chair). Visual and auditory indicators show whether the chosen response is correct. There is also a Delayed Recognition (DR) subtest after 10 minutes for the MSVT and after 30 minutes for the WMT. The consistency (CNS) between the IR and DR scores is computed, and scores on all three subtests (IR, DR, and CNS) are used as measures of effort based on where each score falls when compared against a prespecified cutoff published in the test manuals as well as compared to known groups and research groups.

For rehabilitation professionals new to the topic of validity assessment, an image from a recent case study (Carone, 2014) of a 9-year-old child who presented for neuropsychological evaluation in an outpatient rehabilitation context (referred by her physiatrist) explains just how easy modern PVTs are if the patient is motivated to do well. Figure 2.1 documents severe bilateral brain tissue loss caused by a chronic hemorrhage in utero. The degree of sustained brain damage was permanent, and the child presented with mental retardation (an extremely low Full Scale IQ of 58 combined with extremely low general adaptive functioning) and

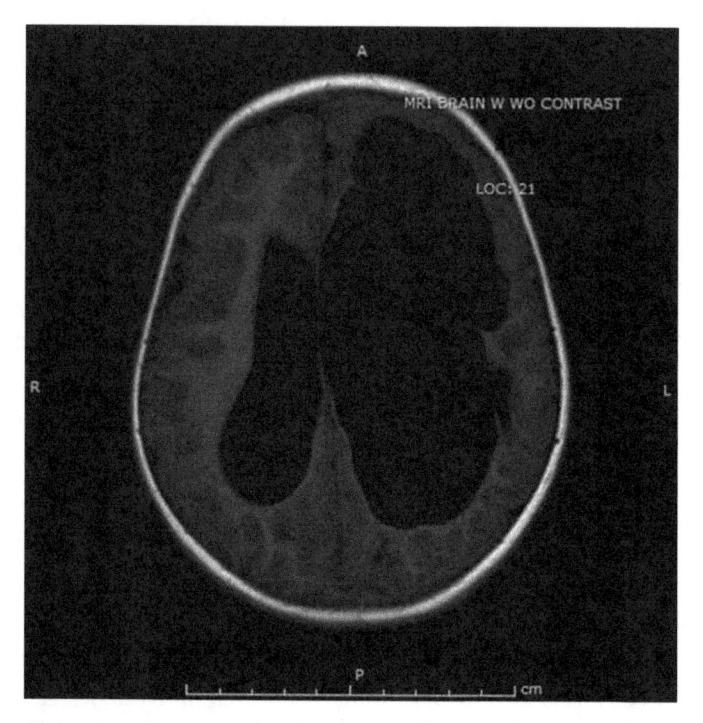

FIGURE 2.1 Brain magnetic resonance imaging at 1 year of age revealing severe bilateral volume loss. From: Carone, D. (2014). Young child with severe brain volume loss easily passes the word memory test and medical symptom validity test: implications for mild TBI. The Clinical Neuropsychologist, 28, 146–162. Reprinted by permission of Taylor & Francis Ltd, http://www.tandfonline.com

chronic epilepsy that was treated with multiple high-dose benzodiazepines. The image was taken at age 1, and the child was evaluated neuropsychologically at age 9. On examination, she was very impulsive and had numerous severe cognitive impairments, including in the areas of new learning and memory (i.e., delayed verbal recall). Despite these severe impairments and severe brain tissue loss, she easily passed both the WMT and the MSVT with perfect to near-perfect scores. The child enjoyed reading, had an interest in words, and had preserved verbal recognition memory, which likely all contributed to her intact performance. The child's performance in the context of her brain MRI, medical history, and cognitive impairments is compelling information to consider when patients with much less severe neurological conditions perform poorly on these tests (see the study in the next paragraph).

When one of us (DC) sought to study the specificity of the MSVT in an outpatient rehabilitation setting, it was done by administering the test to the most neurologically impaired patients available in the context of an outpatient neuropsychological evaluation. These patients were children with moderate to severe brain injury and/or brain disease from heterogeneous conditions such as severe TBI, cerebral palsy, stroke, congenital hydrocephalus, encephalitis, and pervasive developmental disorders. Some children had a combination of multiple severe neurological conditions. Out of 38 such children assessed (average age of 12 and an average education of 5 years), all but two passed the MSVT. Of the two children (5%) who failed the MSVT, one was a child who was responding randomly because she stated that she did not want to be at the evaluation, and the other child was behaving in an obviously oppositional manner. Thus, these children were not false positives but were being accurately classified by the MSVT as providing invalid data. Importantly, these cases show how oppositional test-taking approaches can lead to invalid data and show why validity tests should be used with children in nonmedicolegal settings, as there are other reasons for poor effort besides malingering.

Another interesting aspect of the aforementioned study is what happened when the same test was administered to adults with history of mild TBI or mild head injury with no current or objective evidence of brain injury. The average age for the adults was 37 years, and they had an average of 12 years of education. Thus, the adult group had every conceivable cognitive advantage over the children in terms of neurological and demographic variables but still performed worse than the children. Of the 67 adults tested, 14 (21%) failed the MSVT. The high failure rates among the adults are believed to reflect exaggeration and/or malingering in the context of secondary gain and/or iatrogenesis. Consistent with this interpretation, when the adults and children were asked to rate how difficult the easy subtests of the MSVT were, the adults rated them as much more difficult than the children did. Thus, the study revealed evidence of both performance and symptom invalidity in the adult group, which could not be explained neurologically.

The Test of Memory Malingering (TOMM) (Tombaugh, 1996) is the most commonly used PVT (Martin et al., 2015). This test also uses a forced choice paradigm, but unlike the MSVT and WMT, it is more of a visual-spatial test than a verbal one. Although a "nonverbal" MSVT exists (Green, 2008), it is not truly nonverbal, as the patient needs to name the visual objects presented on the computer. With regard to the TOMM, the patient is presented with 50 line drawings shown for a duration of three seconds each. The patient is then shown each drawing along with an obvious foil (i.e., a drawing that was not previously displayed). Although the presentation is visual-spatial, some verbal encoding likely occurs as patients think of the name of the item shown. The patient is asked to indicate which drawing was previously shown (Trial 1). The patient is then shown the original line drawings a second time followed by another forced-choice phase with foils (Trial 2). Thus, the patient has seen the target stimuli four times altogether, twice independently and twice with foils. If the patient scores below a prespecified cutoff in the test manual on Trial 2, effort is considered poor. If the patient scores above the prespecified cutoff, an optional retention trial can be administered 15 minutes later in which the same forced-choice format is used with the 50 line drawings and foils. Although Trial 1 is considered a learning trial per the test manual, some researchers have published data supporting the use of Trial 1 alone as a PVT because it is generally an easy task (Bauer, O'Bryant, Lynch, McCaffrey, & Fisher, 2007; Denning, 2012; Hilsabeck, Gordon, Hietpas-Wilson, & Zartman, 2011). There is an optional delayed retention trial that can be administered after 15 minutes, in which the 50 target items are shown along new foils. Some clinicians may choose to administer this optional trial on a routine basis based on the premise that some patients trying to appear impaired may instead choose to do so after a delay. However, our experience is that the retention trial is not often administered in clinical practice due to time constraints and (more importantly) because performance on the first two trials is generally highly predictive of performance on the retention trial.

When the TOMM was used in an outpatient rehabilitation treatment setting among acquired brain injury patients, 22% of patients scored below the cutoff despite the nonlitigating nature of the sample (Locke, Smigielski, Powell, & Stevens, 2008). Those who scored below cutoffs on the TOMM performed significantly worse on cognitive tests. Importantly, neither injury severity, time since injury, age, education, depression, nor anxiety was related to TOMM performance. The only factor found to be related to TOMM failure was disability status. Thus, even though an examination in a clinical setting may not be formally classified as medicolegal because it was not referred by an attorney or insurance company (e.g., independent medical evaluation), disability status may still affect performance. For example, patients may perform worse than they are capable on performance-based examinations due to a belief that the evaluation may be used in some way in the future to make disability determinations or maintain disability status.

The Victoria Symptom Validity Test (VSVT) (Slick, Hopp, Strauss, & Thompson, 1997) is a computerized forced-choice test in which 48 five-digit numbers are presented for 5 seconds on the center of the screen. The test is presented to patients as a memory test. The first 16 trials have a 5-second interval, trials 17 to 32 have a 10-second interval, and trials 33 to 48 have a 15-second interval in which the screen goes blank. After each blank screen interval, the patient is shown the target on one side of the screen and a foil on the other side of the screen, and is asked to choose which number was previously shown. Half of the stimuli are easy because the foils (e.g., 21347) share none of the numbers with the target stimuli (e.g., 90865). The other half of the stimuli are labeled "hard" because two of the digits on the foil items are transposed (e.g., 90685), although the task is actually still relatively easy. There are 8 easy and 8 "hard" items for each of the three recognition trials leading to a total of 24 easy items and 24 hard items. Patients are asked to do their best on the test and respond quickly and response times are calculated for the easy and hard items presented as averages and standard deviations.

Poor effort on the VSVT is best detected on the "hard" items based on empirically derived cutoff scores that have been modified over time to improve sensitivity (Jones, 2013) (Macciocchi, Seel, Alderson, & Godsall, 2006). The use of reaction time as an effort measure on the VSVT has some utility, but this is constrained by inadequate sensitivity (Jones, 2013). The VSVT has recently been shown to yield excellent classification accuracy statistics (e.g., sensitivity of .73 and specificity of .98) in detecting poor effort and malingering in mild TBI litigants and military members (Jones, 2013; Silk-Eglit, Lynch, & McCaffrey, 2016). Studies have shown that experimental malingerers and/or compensation-seeking patients score much worse on the VSVT compared to severe TBI patients (Macciocchi et al., 2006), neurological patients with severe amnesia (Slick et al., 2003), children with heterogeneous neurological disorders (Brooks, 2012), and nonlitigating epilepsy surgery candidates (Grote et al., 2000). However, some research with the latter group has shown that working memory deficits, age over 40, and lower intelligence is associated with a higher likelihood of scores falling below the VSVT cutoffs for the "hard" items (Keary et al., 2013; Loring, Lee, & Meador, 2005). In such cases, Keary et al. (2013) suggested using clinical judgment to consider the impact that the these factors may have had on "hard" item scores falling below the cutoff and to consider administering additional PVTs with less of a working memory component before making a final determination about performance validity.

The Word Choice (WC) subest is part of the Advanced Clinical Solutions (NCS Pearson Inc., 2009) package for the Wechsler Scales that helps determine whether patients put forth adequate effort during cognitive testing (Holdnack & Drozdick, 2008; NCS Pearson Inc., 2010). The test is presented as a memory test for common words. In the test, 50 common words are individually presented visually and verbally in a stimulus booklet. Using a dichotomous forced-choice format, the patient must then choose whether the target word was shown or a foil. Each correct response earns one point, leading to a maxiumum total score of 50 points. A cutoff score and norms are available for ages 16 to 69. Obtained scores can be compared to base rates of persons who obtained the same score in the WC normative overall clinical sample as well as various known groups, including persons (1) never exposed to the stimuli, (2) instructed to simulate poor performance, (3) from various neurologic and psychiatric clinical groups, and (4) with similar demographics and intellectual functioning. The WC subtest results can also be readily compared to the results of embedded PVTs from the Wechsler scales. The WC subtest has been shown to have high specificity (90% to 97.8%) and adequate sensitivity (82.6%) when optimal cutoffs scores are used (Barhon et al., 2015; NCS Pearson Inc., 2009). Recently, a time to completion cutoff score was developed for use with the WC subtest and was shown to increase classification accuracy of invalid responding (Erdodi, Tyson, Shahein, et al., 2017) as was the use of critical items (Erdodi, Tyson, Abeare, et al., 2017).

NON-FORCED-CHOICE FREESTANDING PERFORMANCE VALIDITY TESTS

Two popular non-forced-choice PVTs are the *b* Test (Boone, Lu, & Herzberg, 2002a) and the Dot Counting Test (Boone, Lu, & Herzberg, 2002b). The *b* Test examines the total completion time, omission errors, and commission errors on a 15-page task in which the patient is asked to circle all of the lower case b's in the booklet which are interspersed with similar looking letters. The test is used to identify patients suspected of reporting noncredible reading problems (e.g., seeing letters upside down and backward). Cutoff scores and equations combining various performance metrics were created by comparing the performance of clinical groups (such as patients with moderate to severe brain injuries) with real-world suspected malingerers. Per the test manual, sensitivity has been found to be as high as 77%, with specificity of 90% in moderate to severe brain injury populations. The Dot Counting Test works by asking the patient to count grouped dots and ungrouped dots as quickly as possible. Because the grouped dots are more organized, it should not take as long to count them. Thus, poor effort is suspected when the time to count the grouped dots is equal to or greater than the time to count the ungrouped dots.

The test has been shows to have 75% sensitivity and ≥90% specificity in combined clinical groups (e.g., TBI, right and left hemisphere stroke) except for moderate dementia (Boone, Lu, Back, et al., 2002). One non-forced-choice PVT that has generally not proven to be a viable option as a validity measure in its original form is the Fifteen Item Test (FIT) (Rey, 1964). This visual-spatial task involves the presentation of 15 overlearned numbers (e.g., 1, 2, 3), letters (e.g., A, B, C), and shapes (e.g., circle, square, triangle) in five rows of three for 10 seconds. It is emphasized to the patient that *15 different* items will be shown to make the test appear difficult. After the stimulus page is removed, the patient is asked to draw those elements that can be recalled from memory. Production of less than nine items was traditionally considered to reflect feigned amnesia (or poor effort). Although there have been exceptions, numerous studies have shown that the FIT has repeatedly suffered from poor sensitivity (as low as 5%), likely because it is too transparent. That is, most patients appear to be able to detect that it is a simple task. For this reason, sole use of the FIT as a measure of performance validity is grossly insufficient. The FIT has also suffered from poor specificity (as low as 0% in dementia cases and 55% in moderate to severe brain injury cases), likely because a brief exposure with numerous stimuli is actually too challenging for people with severe cognitive impairments. For a review of this literature on the FIT, see Boone, Salazar, Lu, Warner-Chacon, and Razani (2002), who modified the test with a forced-choice recognition memory paradigm to increase sensitivity to 71% and specificity to more than 90%. For ways in which other PVTs help to discriminate between poor effort and genuine severe cognitive impairment in dementia and dementia-like conditions, see chapters 4 and 6.

EMBEDDED PERFORMANCE VALIDITY TESTS

A good example of an embedded PVT is Reliable Digit Span (RDS) (Greiffenstein, Baker, & Gola, 1994) which was originally based on the Digit Span subtest of the Wechsler Adult Intelligence Scale-Third Edition (WAIS-III) (Wechsler, 1997). The RDS is the most commonly used embedded effort test per recent national survey data (Martin et al., 2015). The RDS was designed to assess consistency of responding by summing the longest string of two digits repeated *of the same digit length* without error over two trials in forward and backward conditions. Thus, if a patient correctly repeated a maximum of two consecutive five-digit (5) strings forward and a maximum of two consecutive three-digit (3) number strings backward, the RDS score would be 8 (5 + 3 = 8). This embedded measure has been shown to have high specificity in moderate to severe TBI and high sensitivity in patients with a history of mild TBI who met diagnostic criteria for probable malingering (Mathias, Greve, Bianchini, Houston, & Crouch, 2002). As an example of trade-offs between sensitivity and specificity, the aforementioned study showed that an RDS cutoff score of 5 yields 100% specificity but, because it is rare for patients to score that low, the sensitivity is only 21%, which is not sufficient for clinical use. Increasing the RDS cutoff score to 8 increases the sensitivity to 83% but decreases the specificity to 80%, which is also not sufficient for clinical use. Thus, most clinicians opt for a trade-off by setting the RDS cutoff at 6 or 7, which yields a sensitivity of 38% and 67% respectively and a specificity of 97% and 93%, respectively.

Another way to construct an embedded PVT is to administer a test of cognitive ability and to divide the patients into two groups based on passing or failing performance on validated PVTs. For example, Sawyer, Testa, and Dux (2016) recently used such a procedure to create embedded validity cutoffs for two commonly used tests of learning and memory, the Hopkins Verbal Learning Test-Revised (HVLT-R) (Brandt & Benedict, 2001) and the Brief Visuospatial Memory Test-Revised (BVMT-R) (Benedict, 1997). The HVLT-R is an orally presented list-learning and memory task for 12 words repeated over three trials followed by delayed recall and recognition memory subtests. The BVMT-R is a visual-spatial memory test for six geometric figures presented over three trials followed by delayed recall and recognition memory subtests. Percent retention is calculated on both tests by dividing the delayed recall raw score by the higher raw score of Trial 2 or Trial 3. A discrimination index is also calculated on both tests by subtracting the raw number of recognition memory false alarms from the raw number of recognition memory hits. The authors administered these tests to 109 US military veterans and divided them into a group who passed a combination of all (or all but one) freestanding and embedded PVTs and a group who failed more than one PVT. The authors then used statistical tests (e.g., area under the curve) to show which scores on these two memory tests best discriminated patients in the two PVT groups. The authors found that the HVLT-R Recognition Discrimination Index demonstrated a sensitivity of .53 with specificity of .93 and that the BVMT-R Percent Retention demonstrated sensitivity of .31 with specificity of .92. Study designs such as these with commonly used tests from clinical assessments are of great benefit to clinicians and can serve as a model for embedded validity test construction in other rehabilitation disciplines.

Although most embedded validity assessment measures use a cutoff score, some are based on comparing the patient's pattern of performance to known patterns of performance present in objectively verified cases of brain pathology. A good example of this is analysis of manual motor performance on tests of grip strength, finger-tapping speed, and speeded peg placement. Specifically, Greiffenstein, Baker, and Gola (1996) showed that patients with moderate to severe TBI performed worst on speeded peg placement and best on grip strength. The pattern makes neurological sense because speeded peg placement is the most difficult due to the speeded fine motor integration coordination demands while grip strength is the easiest because it is untimed and does not require coordination. A chronic postconcussion group with normal physical and neurological examinations per board-certified physicians showed essentially the opposite pattern. That is, grip strength performance was the worst (similar to patients with flaccid paralysis), and speeded pegboard placement was much better. Thus, such a pattern of performance is not neurologically based. Patterns of grip strength force have long been recognized by occupational and physical therapists as a way to discriminate between sincere and insincere grip exertions (Hoffmaster, Lech, & Niebuhr, 1993; Schapmire et al., 2002).

Advantages of embedded PVTs are that they do not add extra time to the evaluation and are less prone to coaching because they are not as readily identifiable. The disadvantage of embedded PVTs is that because they are more intrinsically linked to ability measures and were not originally designed to measure effort, they are less specific when used with children, patients with dementia, and some patients with severe neurological conditions. For example, Blaskewitz, Merten, and Kathmann (2008) found that the majority (59%) of healthy children between ages 6 and 11 scored at or below the traditional RDS cutoff used with adults whereas all of them passed the MSVT and the TOMM. Schroeder et al. (2012) noted that clinicians must be cautious in applying RDS as an effort measure in all clinical groups and should be especially cautious when using it in the following groups: stroke, severe memory disorders, mental retardation, borderline intellectual functioning, and patients with English as a second language. We echo these cautions and advise clinicians to only use failure on embedded measures as an indicator of invalid test data when used with patient groups that the test has been validated for and with similar patient groups that have no objective evidence of neuropathology. However, good performance on embedded measures with such groups can be taken as partial evidence of valid test performance.

QUALITATIVE ASSESSMENT OF PERFORMANCE VALIDITY

Qualitative assessment of performance validity involves the detection of atypical behavioral characteristics that are not commonly observed in genuine physical disorders. In some instances the techniques involve asking the patient to perform behavior whereas others involve making observations of spontaneously performed behaviors. One example is qualitative analysis of gait disturbance in which numerous characteristics (e.g., sudden knee buckling without falls) have been shown to distinguish between neurologically based gait disorders and psychogenic/feigned gait disturbances (Baik & Lang, 2007; Lempert, Brandt, Dieterich, & Huppert, 1991). Another example is distraction tests, in which the examiner evaluates whether the performed behavior is present or reduced upon distraction (e.g., the healthcare provider calling the patient's attention to something else), which should not occur in neurological disease. For example, a parkinsonian tremor should remain present when a patient is distracted whereas a psychogenic tremor would resolve upon distraction and resurface under direct observation. Distraction techniques are one of five categories of signs (known as Waddell signs) (Waddell, McCulloch, Kummel, & Venner, 1980) that are *screening* indicators of nonorganic components of reported low back pain. Some of these signs involve behavioral performance (e.g., dramatic overreactions to testing) and others are actually symptom reports (e.g., nonanatomical sensory loss). Cautionary use of Waddell signs includes not using them with patients over age 60, non-Caucasian minorities, or patients with serious spinal pathology or widespread neurological damage (Waddell, 2004).

Distraction tests, other Waddell signs, grip strength consistency, atypical pain behavior, abrupt self-termination, and/or observations of significant discrepancies between behaviors/physiological responses and self-reported symptoms are components of physical effort assessment on most functional capacity evaluations (FCEs). The FCEs are standardized measures of functional abilities designed to assess a worker's ability to perform work-related activities (Gross & Battie, 2005). Although some aspects of validity assessment in FCEs have been found to have scientific merit (Lemstra, Olszynski, & Enright, 2004), others have been criticized for methodological limitations such as poor reliability (King, Tuckwell, & Barrett, 1998; Trippolini et al., 2014). A problem with FCE effort measures is that unlike neuropsychological PVTs, they are generally compared to nonvolunteers or healed workers not seeking compensation (Lemstra et al., 2004). Although performance-based effort measures are an integral aspect of most FCE systems, they are not yet an integral part of standard clinical physical examinations in rehabilitation settings. However, we believe that some form of systematic validity assessment should be used by physiatrists and rehabilitation therapists, recognizing the strengths, weaknesses, and caveats of each particular technique, and referring the patient for a comprehensive assessment with more robust validity measures (e.g., neuropsychological assessment) if there are lingering concerns about the validity of a patient's presentation. See Carone (2013) for a detailed listing of qualitative variables in assessing validity during physical examinations.

Ancillary Issues Regarding Use and Interpretation of Performance Validity Tests

Given that many PVTs involve a memory paradigm and that other domains besides memory are assessed during cognitive evaluations, the question sometimes arises as to whether a PVT is required for *every* possible cognitive domain assessed. Although Boone (2009) stated that this would be the ideal situation, we believe that the practical answer is no. To begin with, there is evidence that poor effort on at least one PVT (the WMT) has a pervasive effect across a wide variety of cognitive domains. Specifically, in a study published in a rehabilitation journal, Green (2007) showed that worse performance on the WMT was related not only to worse performance on verbal *and* visual-spatial memory tests but also to worse performance on tests of intelligence, academic achievement, executive functioning, attention/concentration (auditory and visual-spatial), motor functioning, and even olfactory discrimination. That being said, effort is not always a continuous variable and needs to be evaluated throughout the evaluation, with at least one PVT used early in the evaluation (Bush et al., 2005). Additional time points for PVT use would logically be toward the middle and end of the evaluation.

Recent survey data shows that the average clinical neuropsychologist uses between four and five PVTs, with between one and two being freestanding measures and three being embedded measures (Martin et al., 2015). While such a practice may be transferable to settings in which rehabilitation psychologists are administering a large batteries of tests, it will not transfer to rehabilitation situations (e.g., in settings) in which a brief test battery is used, such as the Repeatable Battery for the Assessment of Neuropsychological Status (RBANS) (Randolph, 1998). In such situations, use of a single freestanding PVT is commonly employed as a validity check along with embedded indicators within the brief test battery being employed, such as the RBANS Effort Index (Novitski, Steele, Karantzoulis, & Randolph, 2012).

Because persons undergoing rehabilitation commonly have sensory and/or motor deficits, the selection, use, and interpretation of PVTs, like ability measures, should take into account such sensory and motor deficits. For example, it would probably be most appropriate for a patient with a visual field defect to be given a verbally based PVT rather than a visually based test of performance validity, or test administration may need to be modified (e.g., oral administration) to ensure that visual stimuli are clearly in the patient's field of vision. In addition, some PVTs allow for modifications of test administration procedures depending on patient limitations. For example, Chafetz, Abrahams, and Kohlmaier (2007) used a combined oral and computer administration (i.e., reading the words for the patient as they are presented on the computer screen) of the MSVT for claimants with low IQ and reading disorders. In some low-functioning patients with significant executive dysfunction and impulsivity, it may be necessary for the examiner to operate the computer mouse for the patient on the MSVT and WMT based on the patient's oral responses. This approach was used by Chafetz and Biondolillo (2012) as well as Carone (2014) and has been approved by the test publisher per the latter authors as an acceptable test modification. It is always important, however, not to modify PVTs in ways that coach the patient to better performance (e.g., warning the patient that they need to do very well on the test; pointing the mouse to the correct answer, making facial expressions or vocalizations indicating the patient is about to choose the wrong response). Providing coaching on PVTs would invalidate the use of these tests and would be inconsistent with ethical practice as it is tantamount to manufacturing data, even if this were done with the best intentions. This is particularly critical in rehabilitation settings where there is a tendency to strongly motivate and encourage patients throughout their rehabilitation course.

It may be tempting to interpret the results of PVTs as reflecting a cognitive construct such as memory. However, with very few exceptions, such as the WMT, which has components (i.e., separate ability subtests) that have been validated at measures of memory, PVTs are not measures of cognitive ability, and the results of such measures should not be used to make statements about the degree of strength or weakness of a patient's cognitive ability. Interpretation of PVT results should be limited to their established purpose; that is, whether a patient approached the evaluation in a valid manner, which would allow the clinician to interpret the results of the ability measures with confidence that they are valid and reflect the constructs of interest. Additionally, caution should be exercised not to overinterpret PVT results in either direction. Interpretation of specific PVT results should be guided by the scientific literature, much of which is published after the initial publication of a test's manual, and determinations regarding performance validity should in most instances be made in conjunction with consideration of multiple factors (e.g., behavioral observations, other test performance, clinical history).

Finally, it may also be tempting to want to use PVTs as therapeutic exercises for patients undergoing cognitive rehabilitation. However, PVTs should never be used for this purpose, because it would not serve the purpose of actually rehabilitating a cognitive ability and could overfamiliarize patients with validity measures during frequent follow-up appointments.

Summary and Conclusions

There is currently a wide range of PVTs available for use in freestanding, embedded, and qualitative formats for making determinations regarding performance validity. Modern freestanding and embedded measures are designed to maximize specificity at the expense of sensitivity. These tests, especially the embedded measures, must be used with acute awareness of their strengths and limitations, particularly when used with young children, dementia patients, and patients with other severe neurological conditions. Qualitative aspects of validity assessment can be used to supplement quantitative PVT use, but should also be used with caution, especially if used in isolation. There is clearly a great need for physiatrists and rehabilitation therapists to develop more reliable and valid measures of effort performance for use in FCEs and clinical settings that are comparable to PVTs used in neuropsychological assessments. This needs to be an area of growing research facilitated by national professional practice associations. This research can be done by using the conceptual frameworks and methodologies in neuropsychological studies, such as validating the measures against known groups, including severely neurologically compromised individuals, to improve specificity.

3   Review of Symptom Validity Assessment Methods

PSYCHOLOGICAL EVALUATIONS USING standardized assessment measures provide a unique and valuable contribution to the understanding and care of rehabilitation patients. For assessment results to reflect the psychological constructs (e.g., depression, anxiety) being assessed, patients must respond in a truthful, valid, and consistent manner. In any rehabilitation context, some patients, for various reasons, will produce results that are not valid representations of the constructs of interest. Where the possibility of secondary gain (e.g., disability benefits, avoidance of responsibility) exists, there is obvious incentive for some patients to skew responses. Other rehabilitation patients, such as those with significant cognitive deficits (e.g., anosognosia or impaired ability to sustain attention), those heavily medicated to treat pain, or those with psychological denial of their problems may unintentionally underestimate psychological difficulties or respond to questions in an inconsistent manner. Clinician judgment alone tends to be inadequate for determining the validity of patient responses and presentations (Dawes, Faust, & Meehl, 1989; Guilmette, 2013). For these reasons, psychometric assessment of symptom validity is an important aspect of the process that clinicians undertake to understand the psychological functioning of rehabilitation patients.

The goal of this chapter is to provide the rehabilitation professional new to validity assessment with a general overview of symptom validity assessment (SVA) methods, examples of some commonly used symptom validity tests (SVTs) with supportive research, and some important issues surrounding the use and interpretation of SVTs. As with coverage of PVTs, we did not aim to provide an exhaustive review of the many different types of SVTs, as this information is available elsewhere (Carone & Bush, 2013; Larrabee, 2005; Morgan & Sweet, 2009). The interested reader is referred to those writings for more detailed information.

Terminology

As noted in the introduction, the term "SVT" is used to refer to a test that evaluates the validity of a patient's responses on self-report scales, as opposed to a PVT, which is used to infer the validity of performance on tests of cognitive and sensory-motor ability. In contrast, symptom validity *assessment* is a more comprehensive process that encompasses all of the ways that the validity of reported symptoms is determined. This process may include symptom validity testing as well as behavioral observations, review of records, interviews of collateral sources, review of surveillance videos or transcripts, and consideration of any other available sources of relevant information. Testing is one part of the assessment process, often an extremely important part, but it is not synonymous with assessment.

There are two types of SVTs that use scores: (1) tests designed for the sole purpose of assessing symptom validity (i.e., freestanding tests) and (2) scales or indices that are components of measures that assess psychological constructs. This chapter describes and provides examples of both types of SVTs. Depending on the practice context and specific patient population, rehabilitation professionals will find the various measures more or less applicable to their individual needs.

Although not covered specifically in this chapter, rehabilitation professionals must also consider *response validity*, which, as described in the Introduction, refers to the accuracy of patient responses to background questions such as education level, work history, substance use history, history of presenting problem, and other background information that may influence case conceptualization, treatment planning, or forensic determinations. Comparing self-reported information with historical records helps to establish response validity.

Symptom Validity Test Paradigms

Symptom validity tests inform clinicians about underreporting and/or overreporting of symptoms. Both freestanding SVTs and scales or indices that are components of more comprehensive measures use similar approaches to assessing validity. These approaches include determining whether (1) an adequate number of responses were generated, (2) the patient responded in a consistent manner to similar items and avoided a fixed response style (e.g., all true or all false), and (3) the patient's responses and scores are consistent with or differ significantly from those of known patient or other normative groups.

SYMPTOM VALIDITY SCALES

It has long been understood by psychologists that determinations about patient effort and validity during psychological evaluations must be made before the results can be interpreted as reflecting the constructs of interest. The Minnesota Multiphasic Personality Inventory (MMPI) in its various formats is the most widely used measure of psychopathology among clinical psychologists and neuropsychologists (Camara, Nathan, & Puente, 2000; Martin, Schroeder, & Odland, 2015; Rabin, Barr, & Burton, 2005). When the first version of the MMPI was published more than 70 years ago (Hathaway & McKinley, 1943), the authors explained that meaningful inferences about the psychological constructs being assessed could not be drawn from the clinical scales without first establishing that the results were reliable and valid for interpretation. Their inclusion of multiple scales to quantify the reliability and validity of the results illustrated the importance of reviewing validity scales as the first step in the interpretation of the data. Extensive clinical use and scientific study since that time have reinforced the necessity of validity assessment and expanded ways to evaluate validity.

Comprehensive Tests of Psychopathology and Personality

Comprehensive measures of emotional states and personality traits developed subsequent to the original MMPI (e.g., Minnesota Multiphasic Personality Inventory-2nd Edition [MMPI-2], MMPI-2 Restructured Form [MMPI-2-RF], Personality Assessment Inventory [PAI], Millon Clinical Multiaxial Inventory, 3rd Edition [MCMI-3]) have also included validity scales with validation studies with various patient populations. There is a tremendous amount of research on these tests and their validity scales, particularly involving the MMPI in its various editions and forms; however, most of the research is not specific to rehabilitation settings or populations. Data from a recent survey of neuropsychologists (Martin et al., 2015) revealed that the MMPI (including MMPI-2, MMPI-2-RF, and unspecified version) is by far the most widely used psychological instrument for assessing symptom validity, with 69.9% of respondents reporting use of the MMPI validity scales, particularly the Response Bias Scale and the Symptom Validity Scale (FBS-r). In contrast, 27.5% reported using the PAI, and 6.9% using the MCMI-III. As a general caution before reviewing some specific SVTs, clinicians should always consider the clinical condition of the patient before interpreting the endorsement of specific symptoms as indicators of exaggeration. For example, a patient with a history of alcoholic blackouts and/or epilepsy will be more likely to validly endorse amnesia for complex behaviors on the Memory Complaints Inventory (discussed later in this chapter) whereas a patient with persisting reported symptoms of concussion would not.

The 338-item MMPI-2-RF, like other versions of the MMPI, has multiple validity measures that assist clinicians with understanding a patient's approach to the test and subsequent response style. The validity scales reflect two general classes of threats to the validity of a protocol: non-content-based invalid responding (consisting of nonresponding, random responding, and fixed responding), and content-based invalid responding (consisting of underreporting or overreporting) (Ben-Porath, 2012).

Non-content-based threats include nonresponding, which is captured by the Cannot Say index and reflects failure to respond to items or responding both "true" and "false" to the same item. Nonresponding artifactually deflates scale scores. It has been recommended that at least 90% of items in a scale be scorable for interpretation to proceed in the standard manner (Ben-Porath, 2013). Dragon, Ben-Porath, and Handel (2012) found that scale score interpretability is significantly compromised if the percentage of scorable responses to the items of a scale falls below 90. If a clinical scale remains elevated in spite of nonresponding, the finding is interpretable; however, the absence of elevation on a scale that has less than 90% scorable responses is uninterpretable. Random and fixed responding to the MMPI-2-RF items is assessed with the Variable Response Inconsistency (VRIN-r) and True Response Inconsistency (TRIN-r) scales respectively. Caution is warranted when VRIN-r or TRIN-r T-scores reach 70, and protocols should be deemed invalid if T-scores on either scale reach or exceed 80.

Content-based threats to protocol validity can be divided into overreported psychopathology and overreported somatic and cognitive complaints, as well as underreporting of common human frailties. The two MMPI-2-RF validity scales that are designed to detect overreporting of psychopathology symptoms are the F-r and Fp-r. Each scale has been found to add incrementally to the other, and both scales have specificities reaching or exceeding .90 based on the cutoffs recommended in the test manual (Ben-Porath, 2013). The Fp-r has been found to be the most effective MMPI-2-RF validity indicator for differentiating between genuine psychopathology and overreporting, with specificity estimates generally well in excess of .90, indicating a false positive rate well below 10%, using a T-score of 100 as the cutoff.

Overreported somatic and cognitive symptoms are assessed with MMPI scales such as the "Fake Bad" Scale (Lees-Haley, English, & Glenn, 1991), now termed

Symptom Validity Scale (but still abbreviated FBS to identify its origin) (Ben-Porath, 2013). For the MMPI-2-RF, a revised version of FBS (FBS-r, also labeled Symptom Validity), the Response Bias Scale (RBS; Gervais, Ben-Porath, Wygant, & Green, 2007), and the F-r and Fs scales provide empirically verified indications of overreported somatic and cognitive complaints (Ben-Porath, 2013). The FBS-r and Fs have been found to be especially informative in the assessment of persons with a history of mild traumatic brain injury, while the RBS adds incremental information in the assessment of exaggerated memory complaints. The F-r contributes as a more general overreporting indicator, given its sensitivity to all three types of overreporting (psychological, somatic, and cognitive).

Regarding underreporting of problems, research with the MMPI-2-RF has been relatively limited, although supportive of the use of its two scales: Uncommon Virtues (L-r) and Adjustment Validity (K-r) (Sellbom & Bagby, 2008). Additional validity scales have also been developed and are commonly employed in some assessment contexts. The Henry-Heilbronner Index (HHI), representing a "pseudosomatic factor," is one such example (Henry, Heilbronner, Algina, & Kaya, 2013; Henry, Heilbronner, Mittenberg, & Enders, 2006). Clinicians who use the MMPI and other comprehensive measures of personality and psychopathology in their rehabilitation practices must be familiar with both the information contained in the test manuals and the scales that were developed after publication of the manuals.

A search of the journal *Rehabilitation Psychology* revealed only one article with "MMPI" or "Minnesota Multiphasic Personality Inventory" in the title since 2000. In contrast, a search for the same title in *The Clinical Neuropsychologist* revealed 97 articles. Of course, some studies published in rehabilitation journals have included use of the MMPI despite it not being the focus of the study. We believe that there is an increased need for the use of omnibus tests of personality and psychopathology in rehabilitation settings, depending on the circumstances of the case.

FREESTANDING SYMPTOM VALIDITY TESTS

Among the tests developed with the primary or sole purpose of assessing symptom validity, Martin et al. (2015) found the Structured Interview of Malingered Symptomatology (SIMS) to be the most commonly used measure, with 10.1% of respondents reporting use of the measure, followed by the Memory Complaints Inventory (MCI), with 6.9% of respondents using that measure. The Structured Interview of Reported Symptoms (SIRS), Miller Forensic Assessment of Symptoms Test (M-FAST), Modified Somatic Perception Questionnaire (MSPQ), Behavior Rating Inventory of Executive Function (BRIEF), and Battery for Health

Improvement-2 (BHI-2) completed the list. We cover the first two of these measures in this section.

Structured Interview of Malingered Symptomatology

The SIMS (Widows & Smith, 2005) is a 75-item true-false measure designed to screen for feigned psychopathology and neuropsychological problems. Five scales target symptoms or conditions thought to be commonly feigned, including Low Intelligence (LI), Affective Disorders (AF), Neurologic Impairment (NI), Psychosis (P), and Amnesia (AM). Initial validation studies using a simulation design demonstrated adequate scale reliability (.80 to .88) and total score classification accuracy (cutoff >14; sensitivity = .96; specificity = .88). Subsequent research has suggested that the original cutoff score results in unacceptable false positive rates, and higher cutoff scores (e.g., ≥23) have been recommended (Boone, 2013). A meta-analytic study involving 31 studies (van Impelen, Merckelbach, Jelicic, & Merten, 2014) found (1) support for the measure's accurate discrimination of feigners and honest responders, (2) resilience to coaching, and (3) concern for elevated false positive rates (lower specificity) in some populations (e.g., schizophrenia, intellectual disability).

Memory Complaints Inventory

The MCI (Green, 2004) is a 58-item computer-administered measure of the validity of subjective problems with memory and concentration. The questions comprise nine scales: General Memory Problems (GMP), Numeric Information Problems (NIP), Visuospatial Memory Problems (VSMP), Verbal Memory Problems (VMP), Pain Interferes with Memory (PIM), Memory Interferes with Work (MIW), Impairment of Remote Memory (IRM), Amnesia for Complex Behavior (ACB), and Amnesia for Antisocial Behavior (AAB). The first six scales identify memory complaints that may reflect neurologically based memory problems, while the last three scales reflect memory problems that are more likely to be fabricated or psychogenic in nature (although some implausibility exceptions can exist, such as in cases of temporal lobe epilepsy).

Responses are analyzed by comparing the mean scores of the patient to those of various comparison groups such as those with various levels of traumatic brain injury (TBI) severity, other neurological conditions, psychiatric conditions (e.g., major depressive disorder), and healthy controls. These groups can often be more specifically parsed based on gender and whether members of the group passed or failed a commonly administered PVT—the Word Memory Test (WMT) (Green, Allen, & Astner, 1996). Results can also be compared to groups of individuals who passed or failed the WMT at various performance levels (e.g., mean WMT score of ≤50%, mean WMT score of 51% to 60%). The computer program automatically computes a best fit analysis to determine which groups are the closest match to memory complaints on the first four scales, the next two scales, and the last three scales. A separate Advanced Interpretation Program (Green, 2009) can be used to determine which of 71 comparison groups are the closest match on all of the MCI scales.

As an example of how this information could be used, results from the MCI may show that a patient's responses are most similar to patients with major depressive disorder who fail PVTs and not at all similar to patients with neurological conditions who pass PVTs. Such information would indicate that nonneurological factors are contributing to overreported memory problems. Such results from the MCI would be all the more compelling if independent information showed that the patient had major depressive disorder and/or failed PVTs.

Recent publications on the MCI have come from Armistead-Jehle and colleagues. Specifically, in a study of 1,597 patients with predominantly neurological conditions involved in disability examinations, it was found that there was a general and systematic increase in MCI scores as performance on PVTs decreased (Armistead-Jehle, Gervais, & Green, 2012b). Thus, overreported/exaggerated memory scores are associated with worse effort on performance-based tests, at least in that study. The results also showed that, in those who passed PVTs, subjective memory complaints (as measured by MCI scores) did not significantly correlate with performance on objective memory tests. Thus, subjective memory complaints should not automatically be equated to a neurologically based memory deficit; other factors contributing to memory complaints (e.g., stress, depression, poor sleep, symptom exaggeration, dissimulation) should be considered. In a follow-up study by these same authors with 191 patients not seeking disability who had neurological and/or possible psychiatric conditions, increased MCI scores corresponded to a general decline in PVT performance (Armistead-Jehle, Gervais, & Green, 2012a).

Lastly, a more recent study with 339 active duty military service members with a history of concussion showed that MCI score elevations were more strongly related to elevations on validity tests from omnibus tests of personality and psychopathology than to worse performance on PVTs, consistent with the MCI being a self-report instrument (Armistead-Jehle, Grills, Bieu, & Kulas, 2016). Although a mean MCI score of ≥ 50% had ≥ 90% specificity, the sensitivity was quite low (.16 to .23) for classifying invalid cognitive test performance. Thus, while MCI scores tend to increase as PVT scores decrease, the authors appropriately recommended that the MCI not be used as a PVT substitute due to other factors (e.g., depression) that can lead to overreported memory complaints. Rather, the MCI should be used as it was originally intended, as a measure to assess the validity of self-reported memory complaints.

SYMPTOM VALIDITY SCALES IN BRIEF INSTRUMENTS

Clinicians in rehabilitation settings commonly use brief measures or symptom inventories to clarify and quantify the nature and extent of patients' symptoms. Such measures are typically susceptible to biased responding because few of them have validity scales or indicators. In this section two symptom inventories that have objective indictors of symptom validity are reviewed.

Brief Battery for Health Improvement-2

The 63-item Brief Battery for Health Improvement-2 (BBHI-2; Disorbio & Bruns, 2002) and its 217-item version (Battery for Health Improvement-2; BHI-2) (Bruns & Disorbio, 2003) are designed to provide a multidimensional assessment of validity and biopsychosocial issues in persons undergoing evaluation and treatment in the context of pain and injury. These multiple choice questionnaires can be administered in paper-and-pencil format or via computer. They were normed with a community sample as well as physical medicine and chronic pain patients. There are three validity scales: validity items (random responding), self-disclosure (fake bad—magnify distress), and defensiveness (fake good—minimize distress). In addition to comparison with the community and patient samples and with the validity groups, the instrument compares respondents to five clinical reference groups (head injury/headache, neck injury, upper extremity injury, lower extremity injury, and back injury). Bruns and Disorbio (2014) reported that (1) the BHI-2 and BBHI-2 are especially well suited for assessing patients with injury, chronic pain, or other somatic disorders; (2) the BHI-2 is the only test that can by itself assess all presurgical assessment criteria; and (3) both versions have been accepted as evidence in several US federal court cases. See Bruns and Disorbio (2014) for a more comprehensive overview of the development, strengths, and weaknesses of these measures.

Neurobehavioral Symptom Inventory

The Neurobehavioral Symptom Inventory (NSI; Cicerone & Kalmar, 1995) is a 22-item self-report measure of physical, cognitive, and emotional/behavioral problems that tend to be rather nonspecific in etiology but have been associated with concussion. The measure is in widespread use with military veterans and has been studied extensively in that context in recent years (e.g., Soble et al., 2014). Because it is a self-report measure and is commonly used in secondary gain contexts, the need to clarify valid from invalid responding became evident. Vanderploeg et al. (2014) described the development and validation of the following three validity scales derived from the NSI: (1) unusual items (NIM5), (2) infrequently endorsed items (LOW6), and (3) nonoverlapping items from those two scales combined (Validity-10). Derivation study participants consisted of active duty military personnel undergoing evaluation in the context of possible TBI and rehabilitation patients ($n = 443$), personnel from the Florida National Guard who completed an online postdeployment survey ($n = 3,127$), and national data from the Veterans Affairs TBI evaluation process ($n = 48,175$). Cutoff scores were generated for each of the three scales and the NSI total score. Using the Mild Brain Injury Atypical Symptoms Scale (Cooper, Nelson, Armistead-Jehle, & Bowles, 2011) as the external criterion measure, the following psychometric properties were reported for these scales: NIM5 >12 (sensitivity = .74; specificity = .93), LOW6 >13 (sensitivity = .66; specificity = .91), Validity-10 >22 (sensitivity = .81; specificity = .94), and NSI total score >58 (sensitivity = .79; specificity = .93).

A cross-validation study (Vanderploeg et al., 2014) involving active duty military personnel ($n = 206$) undergoing neuropsychological evaluation in the context of TBI (69% mild), with the PAI Negative Impression Management scale (T > 75) as the external criterion, produced the following classification accuracies of three scales: NIM5 >12 (sensitivity = .48; specificity = .82), LOW6 >13 (sensitivity = .62; specificity = .83), Validity-10 >22 (sensitivity = .61; specificity = .85), and NSI total score >58 (sensitivity = .59; specificity = .84), which was somewhat lower than the in the initial study.

Lange et al. (2015) studied the clinical utility of the three NSI validity scales, also with a population of military personnel undergoing neuropsychological evaluations following TBI and also using the PAI Negative Impression Management scale as the external criterion. They found high sensitivity, specificity, positive predictive power, and negative predictive power for all three scales, with the Validity-10 scale (optimal cutoff ≥19) consistently having the highest overall values (sensitivity=.59, specificity=.89, PPP = .74, NPP = .80). They concluded, "For the majority of people, these findings provide support for the use of the Validity-10 scale as a *screening* tool for possible symptom exaggeration. When scores on the Validity-10 exceed the cutoff score, it is recommended that (a) researchers and clinicians do not interpret responses on the NSI, and (b) clinicians follow up with a more detailed evaluation, using well-validated symptom validity measures" (p. 853). The MMPI-2-RF is an example of a more comprehensive measure with more extensively researched and well-validated symptom validity scales, as previously described.

Qualitative Assessment of Symptom Validity

The qualitative (nonpsychometric) assessment of symptom validity involves the detection of symptoms, symptom patterns, or levels of symptom severity that are not commonly associated with genuine disorders. Qualitative assessment procedures involve (1) behavioral observations, during and outside of testing sessions; (2) record reviews; and (3) interviews of the patient and/or collateral sources of information. The key to establishing symptom validity is consistency (Slick & Sherman, 2013): consistency between symptom reporting, observations, recorded information, information obtained from collateral sources, and the symptoms known to be associated with the established or suspected disorder. The more inconsistencies or discrepancies that are found within or between these various sources of qualitative data, the less likely that the reported symptoms or observed problems are valid. Sometimes, depending on the level of functioning of the patient being evaluated or the evaluation context, standardized symptom validity assessment is not indicated or appropriate. For example, patients who have an established medical basis for being unable to understand or tolerate lengthy and relatively complex procedures would not be administered such measures, and the measures would not be used in clinical settings where multiple demands on patients' time do not allow for a lengthy assessment process. In such instances, qualitative assessment of symptom validity is the preferred and only way of determining whether a patient is presenting in a valid manner. Invalid symptoms may reflect an exaggeration of valid problems or complete fabrication of the problems. The clinician who adopts a multimethod approach to validity assessment is in the best position to make accurate determinations about symptom validity.

Fundamental Truths about Validity and Its Assessment

Bush and Morgan (2012) presented 12 statements that they considered to be fundamental truths about the assessment of symptom validity with veterans. In this section we offer six statements, derived from the original 12, that we consider to be fundamental truths about symptom validity assessment in rehabilitation contexts.

SOME REHABILITATION PATIENTS PRODUCE INVALID ASSESSMENT RESULTS

There is no denying this fact. There are many reasons for invalid presentations, including a factitious disorder, opposition to the evaluation, the presence of clinical factors such as significant cognitive deficits or florid psychotic symptoms, and the pursuit of secondary gain (malingering).

VALIDITY ASSESSMENT IS ESSENTIAL

Knowing whether a patient's symptoms are valid is essential for developing appropriate treatment plans, providing services, and allocating resources in a manner that is beneficial and not harmful.

EMPIRICAL METHODS ARE MORE ACCURATE AND RELIABLE THAN CLINICAL JUDGMENT

Research has demonstrated that although mental health professionals are trained to analyze and interpret human behavior, clinical judgment alone is inadequate for making determinations about honesty and accuracy of patient self report (e.g., Guilmette, 2013).

A MULTIMETHOD APPROACH IS PREFERRED

A convergence of quantitative and qualitative evidence facilitates determinations about symptoms validity. Obtaining information and data from multiple sources strengthens the clinician's ability to arrive at accurate conclusions about whether a patient's symptom report and behavior are valid.

PSYCHOLOGISTS WANT VALID RESULTS

Psychologists want to use their knowledge of human behavior to assist patients and treatment teams in their rehabilitation efforts. Detecting and understanding misleading symptom reporting and presentations can be part of that process, but the preferred application of clinical skills involves assessing and treating valid cognitive, emotional, and behavioral problems.

DECISIONS SHOULD BE BASED ON SCIENCE AND BEST PRACTICES

There are instances in some clinical settings (e.g., some pain management programs, some concussion treatment programs) in which the value of formal validity assessment is minimized or clinicians are encouraged or instructed by healthcare providers, administrators, or supervisors not to use validity assessment methods or not to interpret the results according to established guidelines. Such instances typically occur in contexts in which appropriate use of validity assessment would negatively impact the fiscal health of the program (e.g., insurance companies no longer authorizing treatments and/or diagnostic tests because of invalid examination results). Instead, clinicians may be advised, inappropriately, to rely on subjective impressions or neglect the issue altogether. Best practices, based on a large body of scientific evidence, dictate that clinicians, administrators, and other stakeholders be aware of and sensitive to the complex nature of symptom validity issues, and support appropriate symptom validity assessment and accurate interpretation of findings.

Summary and Conclusions

Symptom validity assessment is important for establishing the clinician's ability to interpret test results as reflecting the constructs of interest, which in turn is needed for the provision of appropriate rehabilitative services. For a variety of reasons, some rehabilitation patients do not respond honestly to test questions or present in a valid manner. When clinicians provide services based on inaccurate information, resources and time are wasted, and the potential exists for the patient to be harmed, certainly not helped, by inappropriate treatment. A multimethod approach to symptom validity assessment that includes SVTs helps clinicians make decisions about the validity of a patient's presentation, which is necessary for guiding treatment.

Multiple empirically based symptom validity scales embedded within comprehensive psychological measures facilitate the interpretation process, but such comprehensive measures require that patients are being evaluated in a context that allows for a lengthy evaluation process. In some contexts or with some patients, use of briefer psychological measures is preferred, and there are some brief measures that have scales or other indicators of symptom validity. In addition, some freestanding SVTs have been developed specifically to aid in the complex validity assessment process. In this chapter we have reviewed a few of the more commonly used symptom validity measures. Some of the measures have been studied fairly extensively with injury and rehabilitation populations, whereas other available and commonly used SVTs have limited data pertaining to patients commonly evaluated and treated in rehabilitation settings. Additional SVTs used more specifically with children are discussed in chapter 6. Given the diversity of rehabilitation practices, clinicians should select the measures that are most appropriate for their specific needs. Continued research in this area is needed and will further enhance the ability of rehabilitation professionals to provide appropriate, beneficial services while maximizing resources.

4   Validity Assessment in Patients with Brain Injury/Disease

VALIDITY ASSESSMENT IS often discussed in the context of diagnoses that are known to be associated with reports of persisting symptoms and/or disability despite few to no objective biomarkers of neurological injury or illness. Common examples include mild traumatic brain injury (MTBI), fibromyalgia, chronic fatigue syndrome, pain disorders, somatic symptom disorders, and alleged neurotoxic disorders (e.g., multiple chemical sensitivity), particularly among those who are litigating or otherwise compensation-seeking (Mittenberg, Patton, Canyock, & Condit, 2002). Such cases often involve disagreements among multiple medical specialists about the etiology of the persisting symptoms. In such cases, validity assessment provides a unique insight into motivational factors (and by extension, psychological factors) that might be contributing to the clinical presentation.

Although validity assessment is important in the aforementioned types of cases, it is a mistake to believe that it should be limited to controversial cases and/or cases involved in litigation. As noted in the consensus conference statement by the American Academy of Clinical Neuropsychology (Heilbronner, Sweet, Morgan, Larrabee, & Millis, 2009), "The assessment of effort and genuine reporting of symptoms is important in all evaluations," as poor effort and response bias could invalidate results "even in a routine clinical context" (p. 1121). Put another way by the National Academy of Neuropsychology (Bush et al., 2005), "Assessment of response validity, as a component of a medically necessary evaluation, is medically necessary" (p. 419). This chapter focuses on validity assessment in patients with brain injury/disease. Although MTBI is covered, so is validity assessment in more severe neurological conditions such as moderate to severe traumatic brain injury (TBI), stroke, epilepsy, multiple sclerosis, and Huntington's disease.

Traumatic Brain Injury

A fundamental tenet about TBI that assists rehabilitation professionals in understanding, assessing, treating, and managing patients is that it is not a unitary concept. That is, rather than conceptualizing TBI as single entity with many common characteristics, it is more appropriately considered as an injury that occurs along a severity spectrum of mild, moderate, and severe. As outlined by McCrea (2008), although there are differences between the moderate and severe end of the TBI spectrum, they are often considered together (i.e., moderate-severe TBI) because, in both, the functional anatomy of the injury is closely associated with subsequent signs and symptoms, recovery time (typically 1 to 5 years; Millis et al., 2001), disability status, and other outcomes. In addition, the presence of moderate and severe TBI is often clearly and objectively documented by emergency responders (e.g., paramedic notes) based on physical and behavioral observations, supplemented by the results of structural neuroimaging findings in the emergency department. By contrast, in MTBI there is often a lack of objective diagnostic information, making the diagnosis much more reliant on subjective symptom reporting. Moreover, although recovery is considered complete in the vast majority of individuals 7 to 10 days after MTBI (McCrea et al., 2009), poor outcomes (e.g., persisting symptom reporting, disability claims) are strongly related to factors other than brain injury such as premorbid/comorbid psychiatric illness (e.g., major depressive disorder, panic disorder), psychosocial stressors (e.g., divorce, abuse history), neurodevelopmental factors (e.g., history of developmental delays), other neurological problems (e.g., seizure disorder), substance abuse (e.g., alcoholism, seeking controlled substance prescriptions), and/or compensation seeking (e.g., litigation).

Although performance validity assessment in psychology owes its beginnings to the assessment of functional sensory disorders (Pankratz, 1979), it is fair to say that it would not have flourished to the degree that it has today if it were not due to the controversy surrounding persisting symptom reporting after MTBI and the readily available comparison groups that moderate to severe TBI patients offered. Clinicians needed an objective way to determine whether MTBI patients were performing in a valid manner, and many performance validity tests (PVTs) were created to meet that need. It has repeatedly been found that neuropsychological test performance is suppressed far more by poor effort than it is by brain injury severity (Green, Rohling, Lees-Haley, & Allen, 2001; Meyers, Volbrecht, Axelrod, & Reinsch-Boothby, 2011;

Rohling & Demakis, 2010). As a result, if the influence of poor effort is not assessed and controlled for, patients with a history of MTBI could misleadingly present as impaired (or paradoxically more impaired) than patients with a history of moderate to severe TBI. National survey data among neuropsychologists shows that patients with a history of MTBI have a higher base rate (41%) of malingering and exaggeration (based on various criteria) than patients with a history of moderate to severe TBI (9%) (Mittenberg et al., 2002). Consistent with this, studies over the decades have repeatedly shown that patients with a history of MTBI perform much worse on various freestanding PVTs than moderate to severe TBI patients do (Binder, 1993; Green, 2007; Green, Iverson, & Allen, 1999; Haber & Fichtenberg, 2006; Sherer et al., 2015) even when adults are compared to children (Carone, 2008).

Patients with moderate to severe TBIs (and other brain pathology) are more likely to score below established cutoffs on embedded PVTs than freestanding PVTs because, unlike the former, embedded PVTs were originally derived from cognitive ability tests. As an example, one study found that whereas no individuals with moderate to severe TBI ($n = 30$) lacking a substantial external incentive for malingering scored below the cutoffs on two freestanding PVTs, two patients scored below the cutoff of 7 or less on commonly used freestanding PVT (Reliable Digit Span; RDS) (Mathias, Greve, Bianchini, Houston, & Crouch, 2002). A recent systematic review of RDS showed that the average specificity of RDS across multiple studies in patients with moderate to severe TBI was 82% for a cutoff of 7 or less but 99% for a cutoff of 6 or less (Schroeder, Twumasi-Ankrah, Baade, & Marshall, 2012) As others have explained, the additional cognitive demands of backward span may be an issue for patients with significant objective neuropathology such as moderate to severe TBI, a finding that illustrates the importance of interpreting PVT scores based on appropriate comparison groups (Heinly, Greve, Bianchini, Love, & Brennan, 2005). While lowered cutoff scores are one way to address the problem of declining specificity on freestanding PVTs in patients with moderate to severe neuropathology, the downside of lowering cutoff scores is that doing so will decrease sensitivity. For example, Mathias et al. (2002) found that the sensitivity to probable malingering with RDS was 67% with a cutoff score of 7 or below but precipitously dropped to 38% by lowering the cutoff score to 6 or less.

Although freestanding PVTs are remarkably insensitive to brain pathology, some patients can score below established cutoffs due to genuine severe cognitive impairment, the likes of which can occur from severe TBI. Thus, when any patient with a severe neurological condition affecting brain functioning scores below established PVT cutoffs, the examiner must determine whether the score is due to poor effort or genuine severe cognitive impairment. Unfortunately, for embedded PVTs and most freestanding PVTs, the examiner must rely on clinical judgment to make this determination. However, there are three freestanding PVTs that use a procedure known as profile analysis to help make this determination, which is possible because these tests include a combination of traditional effort subtests and ability subtests. These tests are the Word Memory Test (WMT) (Green, 2003), the Medical Symptom Validity Test (MSVT) (Green, 2004), and the Non-Verbal MSVT (NV-MSVT) (Green, 2008). The first step of profile analysis is determining whether the difference between the average score on the "hard subtests" (ability subtests) and "easy subtests" (effort subtests) is the same or greater than a prespecified number of points provided in the test manual. If the difference is not greater than the prespecified number, then poor effort is concluded, even if the patient has a severe neurological condition. If (1) the difference is greater than the prespecified number, (2) none of the effort subtest scores are significantly below chance, and (3) the patient has a severe neurological condition that can cause genuine severe cognitive impairment, then the examiner would conclude that the performance likely reflects good effort and valid data. Thus, profile analysis uses both objective criteria and clinical criteria to reduce false positive rates. This profile was originally referred to as the "dementia profile," but to broaden the terminology to apply to patients with other severe neurological conditions (such as severe TBI), Carone (2009) renamed it the "severe impairment profile" (SIP). As Chafetz and Biondolillo (2013) found, patients who malinger can feign the SIP. Importantly, this is why patients who obtain the SIP who do not have a known or suspected severe neurological condition are still classified as putting forth poor effort because they do not have a condition that is severe enough to plausibly cause scores to fall below established cutoffs. Thus, consistent with a theme repeated in this book, clinical context is critical in interpreting PVT scores.

Stroke

Stroke is one of the most common conditions that rehabilitation professionals assess and treat due to the wide-ranging and often long-term sequelae caused by an acute hemorrhagic and/or ischemic vascular disruption (Langhorne, Bernhardt, & Kwakkel, 2011). Due to severe declines in motor functioning (e.g., hemiplegia, spasticity), psychological functioning (e.g., depression), and cognitive functioning (e.g., cerebrovascular dementia), disability is a common outcome after stroke (Wang, Kapellusch, & Garg, 2014). As such, it is not uncommon for stroke patients to be evaluated in a disability-seeking context with physical and cognitive evaluations, which require careful and accurate documentation of impairment, if present (Patel, 2001).

Despite the incidence of stroke in general and the common presence of stroke patients in rehabilitation settings, there has been a paucity of validity assessment studies with this population. This likely stems at least in part from the fact that many stroke survivors pursuing disability have obvious, objectively verifiable deficits that qualify for disability status and benefits. Further, unlike a subgroup of MTBI patients, there is no current controversy regarding a subset of mild stroke patients who report more symptoms and present with more disability than patients who suffered a moderate to severe stroke. Thus, there has been no impetus for researchers to study comparisons between mild versus moderate to severe stroke patients, perhaps because stroke does not commonly occur in litigation contexts. Nonetheless, some studies of validity assessment performance in stroke patients do exist. For example, Heinly et al. (2005) administered RDS to 517 stroke patients considered to have no substantial external incentive to perform poorly. Using an RDS cutoff of 7 or less and 6 or less, specificity was only 56% and 70%, respectively. For this, reason, Schroeder et al. (2012) later concluded that caution should be used when using RDS with stroke patients. Our position is that while RDS can be used as a marker of good effort in stroke patients, it should not be used in isolation to make conclusions about poor effort in stroke patients.

In a recent study, the Test of Memory Malingering (TOMM; see chapter 2 for additional information) (Tombaugh, 1996) was administered to 266 children (ages 5 to 18) with mixed neurological conditions, and 94% achieved passing scores (Ploetz, Mazur-Mosiewicz, Kirkwood, Sherman, & Brooks, 2016). However, of the various patient groups, children with stroke ($n = 37$) had the lowest pass rate (86%). Of the 5 children with stroke who failed the TOMM, one (age 5) was not engaged and scored below chance; another (age 15) scored at chance on multiple PVTs; another (age 7) had autistic-like behavior and extremely low general cognitive functioning; another (age 8) had severe inattention, borderline general cognitive functioning, and was motivated by stickers; and another (age 11) was cooperative but appeared confused and was extremely low functioning. Thus, failures on the TOMM in these patients appear to have reflected poor effort (91% pass rate when excluding true positives) and/or genuine severe cognitive impairment. For this reason, TOMM scores below the cutoffs should be interpreted with great caution in children with severe cognitive impairment, especially if they are very young.

In addition to this cautionary recommendation for the TOMM, completion time on another PVT, the *b* Test (Boone, Lu, & Herzberg, 2002), should not be used as a validity indicator with stroke patients (right or left hemisphere) as this metric fails to differentiate between this condition and suspected malingering (Boone, 2000). For example, poor performance on this test could be cause by left neglect in right hemisphere stroke patients. However, the number of omission and commission errors on the *b* Test discriminates well between suspected malingerers and left hemisphere stroke patients. Thus, until further evidence emerges, the *b* Test should not be used with right hemisphere stroke patients. Regarding SVTs, the MMPI-2 validity scales have been found to have good specificity in stroke patients ($n = 52$) with regard to the detection of cognitive malingering (based on comparing extreme scores with performance on PVTs) (Greve, Bianchini, Love, Brennan, & Heinly, 2006).

Rehabilitation healthcare professionals should also be aware of "psychogenic pseudostroke," which is an umbrella term used to describe a spectrum of nonorganic, acute, stroke-like presentations, including malingering, factitious disorder, conversion disorder, and functional (i.e., psychiatric) presentations (Behrouz & Benbadis, 2014). Such psychogenic presentations can range from reported mild sensory loss to apparent paralysis (known as psychogenic paralysis). The two main features of psychogenic neurological presentations are inconsistency and absence of objective signs of disease (Behrouz & Benbadis, 2014). Physiatrists and physical therapists can play an important role in situations where psychogenic pseudostroke is considered by evaluating physical motor effort. This includes assessing for the presence of the Hoover sign (not exerting downward pressure in the strong leg when asked to raise the reported weak leg while lying supine; exerting downward pressure in the reported weak leg when asked to raise the other leg); astasia-abasia (staggered gait, appearing to be at risk of falling, but not actually falling or getting injured); dragging a reported weak leg (as opposed to genuine hemiparetic gait with an outward circular movement of the affected leg); splitting of the midline (reporting sensory loss in the middle of the forehead, which is not consistent with neurological sensory distribution patterns); and intermittent motor effort (Kaufman, 2006; Stone, Carson, & Sharpe, 2005).

Epilepsy

Epilepsy is a chronic disorder characterized by recurring seizures. Epilepsy can exist as an isolated neurological condition, can be caused by other neurological conditions (e.g., brain tumors, severe TBI), or can be comorbid with other neurological/medical conditions that are the focus of rehabilitation efforts. Epilepsy can be a disabling condition depending on the severity and frequency of seizure activity, medication side effects, and the degree of cognitive and psychiatric comorbidity (Specht, Coban, Bien, & May, 2015). Interdisciplinary rehabilitation therapies are important aspects of epilepsy management, especially after epilepsy surgery (Clerico, 1989; Mazur-Mosiewicz et al., 2015; Sung, Muller, Jones, & Chan, 2014). In addition, some medications that are needed for management of seizure disorders can have adverse cognitive effects.

Obtaining valid data in epilepsy is critical, particularly in presurgical cases and evaluations for disability determinations. As noted in chapter 2, nonlitigating epilepsy surgery candidates have been shown to perform well on the Victoria Symptom Validity Test (VSVT) (Grote et al., 2000; Slick, Hopp, Strauss, & Thompson, 1997), although other investigators have shown that in some epilepsy patients working memory deficits, age over 40, and lower intelligence are associated with a higher likelihood of scores falling below the VSVT cutoffs for the "hard" items (Keary et al., 2013; Loring, Lee, & Meador, 2005). Other researchers found that 90% of children with epilepsy pass the TOMM but that caution should be used when administering the test to patients with very low IQ, especially if behavioral problems are also present and if ongoing interictal epileptiform activity that can disrupt attention is present (MacAllister, Nakhutina, Bender, Karantzoulis, & Carlson, 2009). Similar findings (96% pass rate on the TOMM) with pediatric epilepsy patients were observed by Ploetz et al. (2016).

Due to the risk of false positive in some epilepsy patients, it is very important for clinicians to use PVTs that can distinguish between PVT failure due to poor effort versus genuine severe cognitive impairment, particularly in a condition in which the temporal lobe(s) are often damaged and dysfunctional, given the important role of the hippocampus in memory. Research has recently shown that the SIP on the WMT was valuable in identifying epilepsy patients with severe memory loss who perform below established WMT cutoffs (Eichstaedt et al., 2014). Such patients were classified as good effort in the context of severe impairment. Consecutive case series data with the VSVT and TOMM show the ease with which these PVTs can be passed by children with neurological conditions such as epilepsy or stroke (Brooks, 2012). Case study data has been presented in children with epilepsy and other co-morbid neurologic conditions (e.g., stroke, severe brain tissue loss, mental retardation), showing the ease with which the MSVT and WMT can be passed, even when there has been removal of the left anterior hippocampus and parahippocampal gyri (Carone, 2014; Carone, Green, & Drane, 2014).

Many more patients with psychogenic nonepileptic seizures (PNES) put forth poor effort on cognitive evaluations compared to patients with epileptic seizures (Drane et al., 2006). Specifically, a striking 51% of patients with PNES failed the WMT compared to only 8% of the epileptic seizure group. The authors concluded that previously ascribed "cognitive impairment" in the PNES group appears to be due to motivational factors as opposed to verifiable neuropathology. This is yet another of many examples in which patients with less (or no) verifiable neuropathology perform significantly worse on PVTs that patients with significant neuropathology. The examples of PNES and psychogenic pseudostroke highlight how genuine neurological illnesses can be mimicked by psychological factors and/or compromised effort.

Multiple Sclerosis

Multiple sclerosis (MS) is a demyelinating condition of the brain and/or spine that causes physical limitations (e.g., sensorimotor abnormalities, fatigue), cognitive impairment (e.g., processing speed slowing and episodic memory problems), and/or psychological dysfunction (e.g., depression) that can lead to limitations with functioning, including work disability (Benedict & Zivadinov, 2011; Jones, Pike, Marshall, & Ye, 2016). As some forms of MS are known for having fluctuating courses, accurate monitoring of functioning over time is especially important. Disability is such a prominent issue in MS assessment and care that a specific scale (Expanded Disability Status Scale; EDSS) based on the results of a neurological examination (which includes assessment of cognitive functioning) and clinical judgment (Kurtzke, 1983) is widely used to monitor it over time. The EDSS scores range from 0 (normal) to 10 (death). Another common measure of functioning in MS patients is the Multiple Sclerosis Functional Composite, which measures walking speed, fine motor functioning (i.e., speeded peg placement), and cognitive functioning (i.e., auditory working memory) (Fischer, Rudick, Cutter, & Reingold, 1999). Thus, ratings of overall functioning and disability in MS are highly dependent on performance-related metrics, as well as the results of neuropsychological evaluations, which are recommended as a routine part of the clinical evaluation of MS patients (Korakas & Tsolaki, 2016). Multiple sclerosis patients have frequent interactions with rehabilitation professionals, with the effectiveness of these interventions ranging from high (i.e., physical therapy) to low (i.e., psychological interventions, occupational therapy strategies) (Khan & Amatya, 2016).

A question that would seem to arise naturally is, how much does patient effort impact the assessment of functioning, disability, and treatment in MS? However, this question has received surprisingly little attention in the published literature. In fact, in what appears to be the first published study on performance validity testing in MS patients ($n = 40$), these patients were actually not the primary focus of the study (van der Werf, Prins, Jongen, van der Meer, & Bleijenberg, 2000). Rather, the MS patients were used as a comparison group for a group of patients with prominent cognitive complaints without a diagnosis ($n = 67$). Both groups were matched on gender, education, and age. These comparison group patients were classified as having chronic fatigue syndrome (CFS), which is a medically unexplained condition characterized by severe and disabling fatigue along with other nonspecific symptoms such as *self-reported* impairment in concentration and short-term memory (Fukuda et al., 1994). The study was performed in the Netherlands, which may be why the PVT selected was the Amsterdam Short-Term Memory Test (ASTMT) (Schagen, Schmand, de Sterke, & Lindeboom, 1997). This test involves asking the examinee to read aloud and remember five words from a single category, perform a simple arithmetic task, and then select from a new page which three words they were shown previously out of five choices (three target words and two foils). The total number of words recognized correctly is the total score. The average EDSS score of the MS patients was 4.1, which is a relatively severe degree of disability. The results showed that 30% of the CFS patients scored below the cutoff on the ASTMT, which was about double the rate of failure in the MS patients (16%). Moreover, whereas 25% of CFS patients scored above a raw score of 16 on a commonly used depression checklist, only 3% of MS patients scored above 16 (upper end of mild) out of 63 points. Thus, the findings paralleled what has been repeatedly observed in performance validity assessment research with TBI patients, in that patient groups with more objective signs of neuropathology and less reported psychiatric distress performed significantly better on PVTs than those with no (or few) objective signs of neuropathology and more reported psychiatric distress.

The authors of the aforementioned study noted that the results cast doubt on the degree that abnormal cognitive test scores can be interpreted as a sign of neurological impairment when there is no other documented evidence of neurological impairment, and they mentioned the iatrogenic harm that can result in doing so. The authors discussed several possible explanations for PVT failure in CFS patients, including excessive stress when confronted with a memory test given their high degree of memory complaints, fear of failure, attempts to make their problems more noticeable for fear their problems will go unnoticed, and adapting behavior to disease expectations (given that cognitive problems are part of the CFS diagnostic criteria). While these factors may have played a role, the disability-seeking status of the patient groups is unknown and could have also played a role in the results for both patient groups. Given that the upper range EDSS score in the MS patients was 6.5 (severe disability), it is possible that severe cognitive impairment could have contributed to some scores below the established ASTMT cutoffs. Without comprehensive neuropsychological assessment results and a PVT that incorporates profile analysis, it is impossible to determine the degree to which genuine cognitive impairment could have lowered the ASTMT scores.

In another case study from outside of the United States (France), a litigating patient with progressive MS scored well below the cutoffs on two very easy PVTs: the Fifteen-Item Test (raw score = 3/15; cutoff score = 10) and the 21-Item Test (Bayard, Adnet Bonte, Nibbio, & Moroni, 2007). See chapter 2 for a discussion of the

Fifteen-Item Test. The 21-Item Test (Iverson, Franzen, & McCracken, 1991) is a screening measure of performance validity with low sensitivity and high specificity that uses a two-item forced-choice recognition paradigm. The PVT scores of the MS patient on these relatively insensitive PVTs were worse than patients with Alzheimer's disease. The authors concluded that the case was unequivocal proof that malingering can co-occur in patients evaluated in litigious contexts who have well-documented neuropathology. Binder (1992) concluded that a man with a possible diagnosis of MS (despite two normal neurological examinations) was malingering on neuropsychological testing based on the presence of moderate to severely low scores and failure on two PVTs in the context of a Social Security Disability Insurance application. It has also been noted that in a diagnostic neurological evaluation for MS, malingering and conversion disorder should be considered in the context of a patient presenting with a constellation of symptoms, questionable objective findings, and normal results from magnetic resonance imaging, cerebrospinal fluid studies, and evoked potentials (Fadil, Kelley, & Gonzalez-Toledo, 2007). While we agree with this recommendation, caution and detailed evaluations are needed before such conclusions are made.

In the only published study using PVTs with MS patients in the United States, the VSVT was administered to 507 patients with MS (Suchy, Chelune, Franchow, & Thorgusen, 2012). The purpose of the study was not to assess performance validity in MS but to determine whether confronting patients about invalid performance affected the results when the VSVT was readministered. Of these, 56 (11%) had invalid performance on the VSVT. Those with invalid performance had higher scores (mean = 23/63, moderate elevation) on a commonly used depression checklist than those with valid performance (mean = 17/63, mild elevation). Whether this reflects a true increase in depression in the nonvalid group or overreporting of depressive symptoms is unknown because no symptom validity tests were used. The authors suggested that poor effort in this sample could have been due to a "cry for help" rather than a conscious attempt to deceive. However, without proper contextual information (e.g., percentage of patients who failed while seeking disability, symptom validity performance, established psychiatric diagnoses, treatment-seeking compliance history), it is impossible to make attributions in this regard. None of this information was presented in the study. The authors also suggested that the MS patients may have performed invalidly as a way to communicate their "invisible" symptom of fatigue to the examiner. However, we do not believe this is a plausible explanation, because patients can indeed be visibly fatigued and often inform examiners when they feel fatigued.

Of the MS patients who failed the VSVT in the aforementioned study, half were confronted about providing insufficient effort immediately after the test was failed, and the other half were not confronted. The confrontation involved reminding the patients to put forth full effort and that a previously administered test showed questionable effort and needed to be repeated. The VSVT was then readministered, making it fairly obvious that it was the PVT despite the authors' later admonition against identifying specific PVTs to patients, linking the confrontation to a specific test, and avoiding referring to tests of effort or performance validity. The findings showed that confrontation resulted in significantly improved VSVT scores (i.e., to the valid range in about two-thirds of patients) and that the effect generalized to tests of memory functioning. The authors' concluded that intervening after nonvalid PVT results increases the likelihood of obtaining valid results.

Recent survey data (Martin, Schroeder, & Odland, 2015) revealed that intervening after nonvalid PVT results is an approach used by a minority of neuropsychologists. Confronting patients about failed performance validity testing during the assessment is an approach that we strongly advise against for two main reasons. First, validity tests were designed to determine the validity of obtained data and not as a tool to influence the assessment results. Second, such confrontations would be expected to help patients more easily identify PVTs, which can compromise future evaluations with the patient or other individuals with whom the patient communicates.

Huntington Disease

Huntington disease (HD) is a genetic and neurodegenerative movement disorder that also results in psychiatric problems and cognitive impairment (Ross & Tabrizi, 2011). The age of onset is typically in the mid-30s to early 40s, but onset at an earlier or later age can occur. The disease is devastating and always eventually becomes disabling, particularly due to progressive deterioration of motor functions and cognition (Ross, Pantelyat, Kogan, & Brandt, 2014), the latter of which can result in a subcortical dementia syndrome (Montoya, Price, Menear, & Lepage, 2006). As a result, patients with HD sometimes undergo cognitive evaluations to clarify their cognitive status. There is no cure for HD, but some patients with HD undergo multidisciplinary rehabilitation efforts in an attempt to improve cognitive functioning, depression, functional capacity, and quality of life (Cruickshank et al., 2015).

At the time of this writing, there has only been one published study of performance validity assessment in HD (Sieck, Smith, Duff, Paulsen, & Beglinger, 2013). The study involved 121 nonlitigating patients with HD, all of whom were administered the Repeatable Battery for the Assessment of Neuropsychological Status (RBANS) (Randolph, 1998). The RBANS is a cognitive screening test used by both neuropsychologists and rehabilitation psychologists. The RBANS contains

12 subtests that yield five index scores in the areas of attention, language, visuospatial/constructional, immediate memory, and delayed memory. It is particularly well suited for rehabilitation contexts due to its brevity and ease of administration. There are two embedded effort measures within the RBANS. The first is known as the Effort Index (EI), which is derived from applying cut scores based on the combined weighted scores of two subtests (Digit Span and List Recognition) known to be relatively resistant to cognitive dysfunction (Silverberg, Wertheimer, & Fichtenberg, 2007). An Effort Scale (ES) was later developed which is derived from a formula that takes into account the performance on five RBANS subtests (Digit Span, List Recognition, List Recall, Story Recall, and Figure Recall) to help identify poor effort (via application of a cutoff score) among patients with memory disorders, which was a weakness with the EI (Novitski, Steele, Karantzoulis, & Randolph, 2012). The formula accounts for the expected pattern of memory decline in most amnestic disorders, in which free recall declines more prominently than recognition memory, unlike most patients who exhibit poor effort on testing. While the ES results in fewer false positives than the EI, the authors only recommend its use in cases where there is low performance on the List Recognition and Digit Span subtests and when there is a question as to whether this was due to poor effort or genuine cognitive impairment. They suggested that additional PVTs be used to clarify the findings in most cases. Thus, the EI and ES should be viewed as performance validity screening measures. See chapter 6 for more detailed information on use of the RBANS effort measures in geriatric patients.

Sieck et al. (2013) found that only 30% of HD patients passed the ES. The authors attributed this high failure rate to the presence of greater attention deficits and better free recall than the ES was designed for (e.g., Alzheimer disease patients). In contrast to the ES findings, the study found that that 82% passed the EI. A subsample of HD patients ($n = 36$) was administered the TOMM, which 92% passed. The authors concluded that the ES may not be a well-suited PVT for HD patients, whereas the EI and TOMM were more useful PVTs with HD patients, particularly for those with mild to moderate cognitive impairment. Although the authors could not exclude the possibility that low PVT scores were due to invalid performance in some patients, they found that failure on the EI and TOMM was associated with more disease-related symptoms (e.g., motor impairment), worse adaptive functioning, and greater amounts of cognitive impairment. Because of this, the authors cautioned against the use of these measures in HD patients who have to severe motor and cognitive impairment (e.g., RBANS Total standard score below 65).

The study by Sieck et al. (2013) contains a number of important points for rehabilitation professionals who are new to validity assessment. First, the study highlights the importance of staying up to date with an evolving research literature to ensure that validity tests are used with appropriate populations to avoid presumed false positive classifications of poor effort. Second, the study shows that modified PVTs should not automatically be considered to be better than their predecessors with all populations. Third, the study demonstrates a prominent weakness with the use of embedded PVTs with patients who have severe cognitive impairment in that doing so increases the risk of false positives. While this risk also occurs with some freestanding PVTs (including the TOMM) when used with patients who have severe cognitive impairment, that risk is mitigated by using freestanding PVTs that incorporate profile analysis to specifically distinguish between low PVT scores due to invalid performance from low PVT scores caused by genuine cognitive impairment. It is partly for this reason that Sieck et al. (2013) suggested, with patients who have moderate to severe cognitive impairment, using tests such as the MSVT, which has been validated as a PVT in dementia cases (see chapter 6).

Conclusions and Future Directions

Whether it is a comparison of MTBI with moderate to severe TBI, CFS with MS, or PNES with epileptic seizures, the literature consistently shows that patients with less (or no) verifiable neuropathology perform significantly worse on PVTs that patients with significant neuropathology. Although most patients with significant neuropathology can pass PVTs, the pass rate depends on the type of PVT that was selected for the particular condition, with embedded PVTs having more false positives than freestanding PVTs. Not all failures on PVTs in patients with significant neuropathology are false positives, however, and for this reason it is important for psychologists to use PVTs that employ profile analysis so PVT failure due to poor effort can be distinguished from PVT failure due to genuine severe cognitive impairment. However, there is a strong need for the development of more PVTs that incorporate profile analysis. In addition, there is a significant need to expand validity assessment research beyond TBI, with more studies specifically focused on performance and symptom validity in non-TBI-related neurological disorders and to use adequate sample sizes.

5 Validity Assessment in Rehabilitation Patients without Brain Disorders

MUCH OF THE research and application of symptom and performance validity assessment has focused on memory problems, which are commonly associated with injuries and illnesses involving the brain. However, problems with memory and other cognitive abilities are nonspecific and are often experienced by noninjured community-dwelling persons as well as patients with wide-ranging medical problems or psychiatric disorders (Arnett, 2013; Johnson, 2008; Lees-Haley & Brown, 1993; Putnam & Millis, 1994). Related factors such as fatigue, pain, medications, and/or litigation can also affect actual or perceived cognitive functioning, immediately or long after an event that causes physical and/or psychological trauma. For example, Lees-Haley et al. (2001) found that 51% of their sample of litigating individuals without brain injuries felt dazed immediately after the trauma, and 65% felt confused. In addition, Lees-Haley and Brown (1993) found that 62% of outpatient family practice patients experience headaches, and 20% report having memory problems. The physical (e.g., fatigue, dizzy spells), emotional (e.g., anger, impatience), and cognitive (e.g., memory, concentration) symptoms that are commonly associated with brain trauma also occur frequently in the normal population (Putnam & Millis, 1994). These symptoms increase in relation to stress, even for individuals without brain trauma (Gouvier et al., 1992), and the time during which patients undergo rehabilitation can be stressful for many patients.

Reported symptoms or test results that are atypical or of a severity that is out of proportion to that which typically results from a given condition need to be understood so that accurate diagnoses can be made, appropriate interventions implemented, and resources allocated appropriately (as well as the converse—avoidance of unneeded treatments and allocation of resources). A variety of environmental and patient factors can compromise the validity of psychological assessment results in rehabilitation patients (Bush & Rush, in press). In outpatient contexts, cell phones can be a disruptive and distracting presence. In inpatient settings, other patients, family members, or staff can be distracting. In any context, factors such as temperature, lighting, and extraneous noise can have an effect on the patient's performance and invalidate test results; therefore, they should be controlled to the extent possible in a manner that is conducive to the assessment process. In addition, situational patient factors such as severe emotional distress, hunger, or the need to use a restroom can affect the patient's ability to focus on assessment questions, instructions, or tasks. To facilitate a valid assessment process, it is important for clinicians to check with patients about these issues prior to beginning the assessment, with instructions to patients to inform the clinician if problems along these lines arise (Bush & Rush, in press). It is also important for clinicians not to retrospectively use these factors to explain failed validity test performance when no evidence exists to support such an explanation.

It has been found that despite training in assessing human behavior and confidence in the ability to do so, psychologists are not particularly good at determining whether patients put forth valid effort when a formal validity assessment approach has not been employed (Guilmette, 2013). For this reason, more than a decade ago the National Academy of Neuropsychology took the position that formal, quantitative assessment of symptom and performance validity should be a component of medically necessary assessments of cognitive and sensorimotor functions (Bush et al., 2005), and other professional organizations followed suit. As a result, Bush and Rush (in press) noted that the list of rehabilitation assessment competencies, reflecting the breadth of assessment knowledge and skill required of rehabilitation psychologists, which was established by the American Board of Rehabilitation Psychology (ABRP) and posted on its website, is incomplete, in part in its omission of the assessment of symptom and performance validity. By adding to other publications on validity assessment, it is hoped that this chapter further reinforces the importance of a formal, multimethod approach to validity assessment that includes psychometric measures with rehabilitation populations that are experiencing problems other than brain injury or illness.

Pain Disorders and Fatigue

Physical pain and fatigue are commonly experienced, individually or in combination, by patients undergoing rehabilitation. The subjective nature of the problems makes them easy to exaggerate, intentionally or unintentionally, without being detected. Understanding the possibility of symptom exaggeration and the potential impact of these problems on cognitive test performance is important for rehabilitation professionals.

PAIN

Physical pain is experienced by many patients who are receiving rehabilitative services. Acute musculoskeletal injuries, orthopedic procedures, burn injuries and associated care, and other conditions for which patients undergo rehabilitation can cause considerable pain. Such pain, which is certainly valid, can adversely affect performance on cognitive tests and distract patients from responding accurately and consistently to questions about psychological functioning, rendering the results an invalid reflection of the underlying construct.

In contrast to acute pain, chronic nonmalignant pain (including pain-related disability) is a more complex, multifaceted condition that involves psychological factors (Dersh et al., 2001; Etherton, 2014; Linton, 2000) and can be influenced by the pursuit of compensation (Gatchel & Gardia, 1999; Rohling et al., 1995). Chronic pain is defined as pain of at least three months' duration that has persisted beyond expected healing time, consists of both unpleasant sensory and emotional qualities, whether or not identifiable organic pathology is present (International Association for the Study of Pain Subcommittee on Classification, 1986), and is remarkably impervious medical therapies (McCracken & Thompson, 2012).

Exaggeration or fabrication of pain occurs in the pursuit of secondary financial gain as well as pain medication, and the lack of objective markers or measures of pain make it difficult to confirm or rule out. Greve et al. (2009b) found that malingered pain is present in a sizable minority (20% to 50%) of patients with chronic pain undergoing evaluation in the context of potentially compensable injuries. Prescribing clinicians are left with the challenging task of balancing the risk of prescribing opioids or other medications when they are not really needed with the risk of not treating or undertreating a valid pain disorder (Bannwarth, 1999; Portenoy, 1996).

Unfortunately, the assessment of pain validity has been quite challenging. Chronic pain is a highly confounded condition, because those with chronic pain do not only experience pain but also commonly experience depression, anxiety, fatigue, sleep problems, comorbid medical conditions, cognitive difficulties, and the effects of medications (McCracken & Thompson, 2012). To assist in determining valid pain presentations from invalid presentations, a large number of methods that are purportedly sensitive to malingered pain have been developed (Fishbain, Cutler, Rosomoff, & Rosomoff, 1999; Lechner, Bradbury, & Bradley, 1998); however, Fishbain et al. (1999) concluded that as of the time of their literature review, there were no reliable methods for assessing malingered pain. Bianchini, Greve, and Glynn (2005), building on the methodology proposed by Slick, Sherman, and Iverson (1999) for malingered neurocognitive dysfunction, outlined an approach to validity assessment with pain patients that can help clinicians make correct determinations about the validity of reported pain and malingered pain-related disability (MPRD). Probabilistic language (e.g., definite, probable, possible) is used. They defined MPRD as "the intentional exaggeration or fabrication of cognitive, emotional, behavioral, or physical dysfunction attributed to pain for the purposes of obtaining financial gain, to avoid work, or to obtain drugs (incentive). They noted, "Discriminating between unconscious and intentional mechanisms (e.g., hysterical conversion reaction vs. malingering) is one of the central questions that must be addressed" (p. 405). Because cognitive symptoms are relatively common among pain patients (Iverson & McCracken, 1997), are sometimes more severe for pain patients than those with neurological injury (Iverson, King, Scott, & Adams, 2001), and are commonly under voluntary control (Gervais, Green, Allen, & Iverson, 2001), intent could be established with significantly below chance performance on a performance validity test (PVT) or with compelling inconsistencies between the way a patient presents when being evaluated compared with when they are not aware of being evaluated. Objective PVT results are also used to help make determinations about probable and possible MPRD.

Research on commonly used symptom validity tests (SVTs) revealed that among the Minnesota Multiphasic Personality Inventory-2nd Edition (MMPI-2) validity scales, the FBS (Fake Bad Scale; now known as the Symptom Validity Scale) has good sensitivity (69%) with excellent specificity (95%) when distinguishing a group of Definite MPRD from a nonmalingering chronic pain group (Bianchini et al., 2008). Similarly, Wygant et al. (2011) found that the MMPI-2 Restructured Form (MMPI-2-RF) symptom validity scale (FBS-r) and infrequent somatic response scale (Fs) exhibited large effect sizes in differentiating disability litigants (60% of whom claimed injuries with persistent pain) who exhibited symptoms of MPRD from litigants with no evidence of noncredible responding. Regarding PVTs, Bianchini et al. recommended comparing pain patients to groups with moderate-severe TBI, because persons with pain disorders would not be expected to perform more poorly than those with a history of significant brain trauma; however, some PVT research with pain populations allows for direct comparisons.

For example, Greve et al. (2009b) studied pain patients' performances on the Test of Memory Malingering (TOMM). For the detection of MPRD, Trial 1 <35, Trial 2 <46, or Retention <46 resulted in sensitivity of 49.5% and specificity of 99%. They provided different cutoff scores at various false positive rates, thus allowing clinicians to choose a cutoff score based on their preferences regarding sensitivity and specificity. In their sample of 118 participants who were deemed not to be malingering pain-related disability, no one achieved a Trial 1 score of less than 40, a Trial 2 score of less than 49, or a Retention score of less than 47. They concluded that the TOMM is highly effective in differentiating malingering from nonmalingering in their sample of pain patients. Because those participants who were deemed not to be malingering had substantial physical pathology but those considered to be malingering had minimal physical pathology, the authors further concluded that TOMM failures at the cutoffs identified in their study were "not likely attributable to the effects of physical injury or the cognitive effects of variables associated with physical injury. Rather such performance should be interpreted as reflecting underperformance related to non-clinical factors" (pp. 18–19). These authors, studying the Portland Digit Recognition Test (PDRT), found that scores higher than the original cutoffs used for the test could be interpreted as reflecting suboptimal performance for pain patients (Greve et al. 2009a). Additionally, Greve et al. (2010) used a criterion (known) groups validation design to study the classification accuracy of Reliable Digit Span (RDS) in a large group of chronic pain patients who were referred for psychological evaluation. They found that, consistent with prior studies examining a wide variety of populations, a score of six or less proved most accurate in differentiating MPRD from pain patients who were deemed non-MPRD.

FIBROMYALGIA AND CHRONIC FATIGUE SYNDROME

Several diagnoses that commonly involve cognitive and other neurological symptoms but have no or few objective biomarkers of pathophysiological origin, such as fibromyalgia and chronic fatigue syndrome (CFS), have previously been combined conceptually with chronic pain for purposes of discussion and described as *medically unexplained symptoms* (e.g., Binder & Campbell, 2004). Noncredible somatic symptoms tend to present as unusual or exaggerated symptom report on self-report measures, underperformance on motor measures, and cognitive deficits that are atypical for bona fide disorders, as well as misrepresentation of pre-illness symptoms and functioning (Heilbronner et al., 2009).

Performance validity research with these populations frequently reveals test scores in ranges that are consistent with suboptimal performance, often much poorer performance than groups of patients with clear evidence of severe neurological injury or illness. For example, Gervais et al. (2001b) found that the mean performance of a group of fibromyalgia patients who were receiving or seeking disability benefits was lower than previously published mean scores of groups with established neurologically based memory impairment; 24% scored below a very conservative cutoff on the Computerized Assessment of Response Bias (CARB), and 30% scored below cutoffs for the Word Memory Test (WMT). Suhr (2003) compared fibromyalgia patients to a group that had various chronic pain disorders and to healthy age-matched controls on the Exaggeration Index of the Auditory Verbal Learning Test-Expanded (later published by Suhr, Gunstad, Greub, & Barrish, 2004) and found that 18% of the fibromyalgia group and 19% of the chronic pain group failed the effort indicator, whereas none of the healthy control group failed the indicator. However, it is unclear from the study whether the subgroup that failed validity tests differed in some meaningful way from the other pain patients in terms of their clinical condition. Iverson et al. (2007), examining the effects of fibromyalgia on TOMM performance, found that TOMM scores were not affected by chronic pain, depression, or both. They reported, "Despite relatively high levels of self-reported depression, chronic pain, and disability, not a single patient failed the TOMM" (p. 532). Johnson-Greene, Brooks, and Ference (2013), examining the PVT performance of persons with fibromyalgia on the WMT, TOMM, and RDS, found that "PVT performance and disability status are associated with exaggeration of non-cognitive symptoms such as pain, sleep, and fatigue in persons with fibromyalgia" (p. 148). They concluded that their study reinforced the importance of performance validity assessment when working with medical populations. Unfortunately, in a review of the literature, Suhr and Spickard (2007) found that of 10 neuropsychological studies of fibromyalgia conducted to that time, only one assessed and controlled for effort. Although neuropsychological deficits in CFS are sometimes believed to result from failure in effort mobilization, Suhr and Spickard (2007), having considered the PVT evidence, suggested that it is the *perception* of required effort (a psychological process) that is at issue, rather than a neurological process.

Very limited research was found specific to PVT performance and CFS. Constant et al. (2011), in their comparison of the cognitive performance of persons with CFS to those with major depressive disorder and healthy controls, examined performance validity using the WMT and some additional experimental PVTs. In their sample of 25 persons with CFS, the mean WMT IR score was 95.84%, and the mean DR score was 94.40%, consistent with adequate effort. Neuropsychological performance of the CFS sample revealed impairments in attention and memory. Similarly, Binder et al. (2001) did not find evidence of suboptimal performance on a forced choice recall measure with a research sample of CFS patients who did not consider themselves to be disabled. In addition, Busichio, Tiersky, DeLuca, and Natelson (2004) administered the TOMM to 34 participants with CFS, and none scored in the range reflecting suboptimal performance. In contrast, van der Werf, Prins, Jongen, van der Meer, and Bleijenberg (2000) did find evidence of suboptimal performance (30% failure rate) on a forced choice recall measure with a clinical sample of CFS patients. Additionally, van der Werf, de Vree, van der Meer, and Bleijenberg (2002) obtained a 23% failure rate on a forced choice recall measure in their sample of patients with CFS. Similar to fibromyalgia, in a review of the literature, Suhr and Spickard (2007) found that of 21 neuropsychological studies of CFS conducted to that time, only three assessed and controlled for effort. Based on their review of the literature, Suhr and Spickard (2007) concluded, "it is necessary to consider the role poor effort plays in neuropsychological assessment of individuals with pain- and fatigue-related medical conditions" (p. 271). "It would be poor clinical practice to ignore the role poor effort may play in such conditions and instead attribute these symptoms solely to disease or injury" (p. 273).

RHEUMATIC DISEASES

Persons with rheumatic diseases such as systemic lupus erythematosus (SLE, lupus), rheumatoid arthritis, and osteoarthritis can come under the care of rehabilitation professionals, including psychologists. Some of these diseases (e.g., osteoarthritis) result from wear and tear on the body, whereas others are caused by problems with the immune system. Pain, fatigue, weakness, and stiffness are common problems associated with these disorders. Neuropsychiatric syndromes are common in persons with SLE. Brey et al. (2002) found that 80% of the first 128 SLE participants admitted to their longitudinal study experienced one or more neurologic and/or psychiatric problems. Headaches, cognitive symptoms, and psychiatric disorders were the most commonly encountered problems. The battery of neuropsychology tests recommended by the American College of Rheumatology (1999) does not include symptom or performance validity measures. Therefore, the very few studies that have quantitatively examined cognitive performance in persons with SLE, including those studies that used the recommended battery, did not assess these important factors (see, for example, Kozora, Arciniegas, Zhang, & West, 2007). Some general or combined pain populations used in PVT studies have almost certainly included persons with rheumatologic diseases, but studies specifically targeting SLE or other rheumatologic diseases were not found.

Given the strong cognitive and emotional comorbidity in this population, clinicians are left with an incomplete understanding of the likely impact of invalid responding and performance by some persons with SLE. We recommend using PVTs when assessing cognitive and motor functions with this population and comparing the PVT results to groups of patients with well-established significant neurological disorders, such as severe TBI, because there is no neurological reason to expect that persons with SLE should be performing more poorly than those with severe TBI. Clearly, more research is needed in this area.

Orthopedic and Spinal Cord Injuries

Despite multiple possible reasons, including litigation and disability claims, for invalid responses and test performance by persons with a history of orthopedic injuries or spinal cord injuries, very little research was found that was specific to these patient populations, particularly in rehabilitation contexts. Gervais, Rohling, Green, and Ford (2004) compared failure rates on three PVTs (WMT, TOMM, CARB) in a large group of disability claimants who presented with nonhead injuries, approximately two-thirds of whom had orthopedic injuries involving the head/jaw, neck, back, or extremities, with the second most common (8.7%) being a combined group of claimants with fibromyalgia or CFS. Thirty-five percent of the claimants failed one or more of the PVTs, with significantly below average scores being rare (0.04%). Twice as many claimants failed the WMT as failed the TOMM and CARB combined. Although we are unaware of any studies specifically designed to assess PVT performance in spinal cord injury patients, Larrabee (2003) found that definite and probable personal injury litigants had significantly higher elevations on MMPI-2 clinical scales 1 (Hypochondriasis), 3 (Hysteria), and 7 (Psychasthenia) compared to patients with spinal cord injuries, chronic pain, multiple sclerosis, and depression.

Psychological Disorders

The assessment of psychopathology is a multifaceted, data-driven process. The validity of reported psychopathology has long been assessed with psychological tests, the most common of which is the MMPI family of tests (Rabin et al., 2005). Clinical psychologists learn to recognize profiles of invalid responding during their education and training. In contrast, it is much less common for practitioners to learn during traditional clinical education and training about the impact of psychiatric disorders on PVT performance. As a result, because problems with concentration and memory are known to be symptoms of multiple psychiatric disorders and to affect performance on neurocognitive tests, some clinicians may be inclined to attribute poor PVT performance to the effects of the psychopathology. Understanding the performance of persons with various psychological disorders on PVTs allows clinicians to make evidence-based decisions about the impact, or lack thereof, of psychopathology on PVT performance. Heilbronner et al. (2009) stated, "Regardless of the specific type of psychopathology, it is incumbent upon the examiner to perform a formal, in-depth diagnostic evaluation. It is the *totality* of the claimant's presentation that should be taken into account when assessing the validity of claims of psychopathology and/or emotional distress" (p. 1112).

Although psychopathology and its impact on functioning exists on a continuum from very mild to very severe, research suggests that, overall, persons with anxiety and depression who are not involved in litigation or pursuing disability benefits perform very well on PVTs (Goldberg, Back-Madruga, & Boone, 2007). In their review of the literature, Goldberg et al. (2007) found that there was no impact of depression on 12 separate performance validity indicators. Similarly, although fewer studies were found, there was no effect of anxiety disorders, obsessive-compulsive disorder, and somatoform disorders on Digit Span variables or TOMM scores. Ashendorf, Constantinou, and McCaffrey (2004) obtained no failures on the TOMM in a sample of 197 community-dwelling older adults with depression or anxiety.

In contrast, Goldberg et al. (2007) found that psychosis was associated with a modest increase in false-positive results on some commonly used PVTs (e.g., WMT, Digit Span variables), particularly for patients with negative symptoms, concentration problems, and lower education levels. They suggested that cutoff scores could be adjusted downward to achieve adequate specificity ($\geq$90%), although sensitivity would be sacrificed. However, these authors found that some PVTs (e.g., TOMM, Victoria Symptom Validity Test [VSVT]) were relatively unaffected and would be preferable for patients with psychotic disorders.

Posttraumatic stress disorder (PTSD) co-occurs in some rehabilitation patients following both military and civilian injuries and illnesses, and acute care experiences themselves have been associated with posttraumatic stress (Brenner et al., 2015; Elliott, McKinley Fien, & Elliott, 2016; Jackson et al., 2016). Cognitive problems are experienced by some patients who are experiencing posttraumatic stress, often co-occurring in patients with a history of TBI (Larsen et al., 2013; Lew et al., 2009). And PTSD is among the fastest growing of compensated medical conditions (Speroff et al., 2012).

Research with Vietnam veterans using the MMPI-2, SIRS (Structured Interview of Reported Symptoms; Rogers, Gillis, Dickens, & Bagby, 1991), and SIMS (Structured Inventory of Malingered Symptomatology; Widows & Smith,

2005) found exaggerated PTSD symptoms to be as high as 53% (e.g., Freeman, Powell, & Kimbrell, 2008). Tolin et al. (2010) found that the MMPI-2 validity scales can accurately detect noncredible responding in veterans undergoing Veterans Administration PTSD evaluations. Specifically, the F (Infrequency), Fb (changes in responding from the first and second half of the test), F-K (F scale raw score minus K scale raw score), FBS, and FPTSD (Infrequency Posttraumatic Stress Disorder) scales and the Meyers Index (which combines seven different MMPI-2 validity scales into a common weighted method of assessing symptom validity; Meyers, Millis, & Volkert, 2002) demonstrated adequate sensitivity, specificity, and efficiency, whereas the Ds-R (Dissimulation Scale-Revised) and M-DFI (Malingering—Discriminant Function Index) performed poorly. Briefer measures that specifically focus on PTSD symptoms (e.g., Trauma Symptom Inventory [TSI], PTSD Checklist-5) have, at best, few validity indicators and minimal research supporting the use of the validity indicators with known groups. Although the TSI has three validity scales, Rubenzer (2009), in his review of a number of measures, concluded that it has scant scientific support for use in determining symptom validity.

Regarding PVT use with PTSD populations, one case study illustrated the value of using the two-alternative forced-choice paradigm with persons pursuing compensation for PTSD (Rosen & Powell, 2003). These authors noted that failure to include PVTs in research into the relationship between PTSD and cognition contaminates the neuropsychological literature and leads to erroneous conclusions about cognitive effects of PTSD. With just one case study in the scientific literature, Goldberg et al. (2007), at the time of their literature review, found no empirical studies examining the effects of posttraumatic stress on PVT performance. Shortly thereafter, Demakis, Gervais, and Rohling (2008) examined both SVTs and PVTs in compensation claimants (e.g., work-related injuries, civil litigation due to motor vehicle collisions) with PTSD symptoms. The PVTs consisted of the WMT, CARB, a California Verbal Learning Test (CVLT) algorithm, and the TOMM. They obtained PVT failure rates ranging from a high of 20% on the WMT to a low of 7% on the TOMM. Overall, 29% of participants failed at least one PVT, and 48% failed at least one SVT. They also found that poor performance on PVTs was not significantly related to invalid responding on SVTs, indicating that performance on these two different types of validity assessment measures is dissociable and reflects different approaches to responding on cognitive and psychological measures. These investigators concluded, "our findings suggest the need for the evaluation of the veracity of both cognitive and psychological complaints from individuals who are being evaluated for PTSD in a forensic context" (p. 890).

A review of the literature in the past 10 years suggests that PVT performance with PTSD populations has not become a major focus of investigation. The WMT includes PTSD comparison groups in its normative data, which is helpful for clinicians who wish to make direct comparisons. It seems reasonable to expect that persons with PTSD will perform in a manner similar to persons with more general anxiety on PVTs; that is, as a group, those not pursing compensation or benefits will perform quite well, while a sizable minority of those pursuing compensation or benefits will perform poorly on PVTs.

SOMATIC SYMPTOM (SOMATOFORM) AND RELATED DISORDERS

Diagnoses that have prominent somatic symptoms that are associated with significant stress and impairment but are disproportionate to or lack an established medical etiology are referred to broadly in the DSM-5 (American Psychiatric Association, 2013) as somatic symptom and related disorders. The specific disorders include somatic symptom disorder (referred to in its prior iteration as somatoform disorder), illness anxiety disorder, conversion disorder (functional neurological symptom disorder; limited to sensory and motor symptoms), psychological factors affecting other medical conditions, factitious disorder, other specified somatic symptoms and related disorder, and unspecified somatic symptom disorder. Due to a relatively high estimated prevalence (approximately 19% for undifferentiated somatoform disorder alone; Creed & Barsky, 2004, Hiller et al., 2006) and a tendency toward a high level of medical care use, persons with such disorders are frequently encountered by rehabilitation professionals. Because neurological symptoms involving sensory and motor problems occur in conversion disorders, it makes intuitive sense that other neurological symptoms, such as cognitive deficits, could also result. However, none of the specific somatic symptom disorders specifically includes cognitive symptoms. To address this omission in the diagnostic nomenclature, Delis and Wetter (2007) proposed the term "cogniform disorder" as a way to classify patients who exhibit excessive cognitive complaints in widespread areas of life, resulting in a conversion-like adoption of the sick role (manifested primarily as cognitive dysfunction) and who do not show sufficient evidence of intentionality to be classified as malingering. Although intuitively appealing, the concept has not achieved widespread clinical acceptance nor resulted in additional published studies.

Lamberty (2008) provided an informative overview of medically unexplained symptoms and somatic symptom disorders, including assessment and treatment issues. He noted that somatization clearly affects patients' reports and experiences of cognitive dysfunction, despite such dysfunction typically not resulting from brain pathology. He further stated, "Somatizing patients can challenge the clinical acumen, patience, and empathy of the neuropsychologist at any stage of the evaluation process" (p. xii). Nevertheless, it is important for clinicians to be familiar with evidence-based management and treatment options so that appropriate services can be provided or appropriate referrals can be made.

Very little research on validity assessment with somatic symptom and related disorders exists (see review by Merten & Merkelbach, 2013), in part due to methodological challenges. Nevertheless, these authors recommended, "When patients present with unusual, atypical, and difficult-to-understand complaints known as dissociative and somatoform disorders or medically unexplained symptoms, clinicians may administer symptom validity tests (SVTs) to determine whether or not the patient exhibits negative response bias" (p. 122).

Research on the MMPI-2-RF with persons who have medical and somatoform (termed "somatic symptom disorders" in the DSM-5) disorders has been promising. Wygant et al. (2009) found the FBS-r and the Fs scales scales to differentiate, with large effects sizes, groups of patients with bona fide medical disorders from participants instructed to feign medical problems in the context of a disability evaluation. Sellbom et al. (2011) compared a group of participants instructed to feign or exaggerate health problems as if they were participating in a disability evaluation for a work-related injury to a group of somatoform patients (87% of whom had pain disorders) and a bona fide medical sample. The study revealed that the MMPI-2-RF validity scales are useful both for detecting noncredible somatic presentations and for differentiating between somatic malingering and somatoform disorders. The FBS-r demonstrated utility in identifying noncredible somatic complaints but not for differentiating the underlying motivation (i.e., intentional malingering vs. psychogenic somatization). The FBS-r is likely to be elevated (e.g., above 70T) with patients who present with noncredible somatic symptoms but must be considered in relation to other validity scales; the Fs and Fp-r (Infrequency Psychopathology Scale-revised) need not to be elevated (i.e., less than 75T) for the elevated FBS-r score to reflect malingering. The Fs scale demonstrated utility in identifying somatic malingering, as well as differentiating both medical and somatoform patients from somatic malingerers. The Fp-r was found to have the best specificity and positive predictive power rates but had unacceptably low sensitivity to justify its use in isolation. The F-r (Infrequency-revised) scale was not found to be helpful in answering questions of somatic malingering. These MMPI-2-RF studies illustrate the value of using measures that assess symptom validity quantitatively. Briefer symptom inventories that lack robust validity scales are unlikely to be of much value in identifying and differentiating noncredible responding and somatoform disorders. Regarding interpretation of invalid SVT results, Merten and Merkelbach (2013) argued, "there is no empirical evidence to suggest that psychological problems may foster SVT failure per se.... Negative response bias allows for only one conclusion: the patient's self-report of symptoms and life history can no longer be taken at face value" (p. 122).

COGNIPHOBIA

Some rehabilitation patients report experiencing the onset or exacerbation of headaches or other neurological symptoms as a result of mental exertion. Fear of developing such symptoms can result in avoidance of mental exertion, which reflects a condition known as *cogniphobia*. This concept parallels the concept of *kinesiophobia*, which is the avoidance of physical activities because of fear that they might induce (nonheadache) pain. Cogniphobia was first proposed in 1998 by Todd, Martelli, and Grayson (1998) as an extension of kinesiophobia to an unreasonable or irrational fear of headache pain or painful reinjury upon cognitive exertion. Subsequent research has revealed that cogniphobia is associated with poorer performance on some cognitive tests, apparently due to putting forth limited effort on the tests in an attempt to avoid the onset or worsening of headaches (Silverberg, Iverson, & Paneka, 2017; Suhr & Spickard, 2012). Silverberg et al. found a significant correlation between higher scores on a cogniphobia scale and worse performance on the MSVT. These authors stated that cogniphobia could have resulted in reduced effort but that other factors (e.g., compensation seeking) could have resulted in both reduced effort and high scores on questionnaires, including the cogniphobia scale. Suhr and Spickard (2012) found that only 6 of 74 undergraduate students reporting frequent headaches failed the WMT, likely because the authors used modified cutoffs rather than published cutoffs. Nevertheless, the authors found a negative correlation between fear/avoidance and cognitive test performance when patients who failed the WMT were removed. Although some of the research on this topic has been conducted with persons who have a history of TBI, the concept of cogniphobia can apply to persons who are experiencing neurological, including cognitive, symptoms from nonneurological causes.

Those who avoid mental exertion have also demonstrated a tendency to avoid physical activity and traumatic stress triggers (Silverberg et al., 2017). These authors suggested that cogniphobia may reflect a broader avoidant coping style. This coping style is sometimes encouraged or reinforced by well-meaning professionals who subscribe to the belief that mental activity should be minimized to avoid triggering neurological symptoms, even months or years following a mild TBI. Unfortunately, this can lead to an iatrogenically induced activity intolerance cascade in which prolonged activity restriction actually worsens outcomes (DiFazio, Silverberg, Kirkwood, Bernier, & Iverson, 2015). Rehabilitation psychologists are likely to encounter patients who have adopted avoidant coping styles and to quantitatively assess their cognition. Because patients with this condition, by definition, tend to limit mental exertion, assessment of performance validity is particularly important.

CASE ILLUSTRATION

A 54-year-old Asian American woman has been receiving physical therapy, massage therapy, acupuncture, chiropractic care, and pain management services in a private outpatient clinic since sustaining three bulging discs (no herniations) in her cervical spine in a motor vehicle collision one year ago. Despite the various therapies, trigger point and epidural injections, and opioid medications, she continues to suffer with considerable pain. Consultation with a spine specialist revealed that surgery is not indicated. She is distraught because of the persisting pain and lack of solutions, so her physiatrist refers her for psychological services.

The rehabilitation psychologist learns during the initial appointment that the patient has very little social support. She is divorced and has no children and only one friend. She was born and raised in the United States, and English is her native language, but her parents live out of state, and they have not been in close contact in years. She graduated from high school and has been working as an administrative assistant for an accountant for 10 years, a job she did not care for but stuck with to pay the bills. She has been unable to return to work and does very little other than attend her therapy and medical appointments. She has been neglecting household chores and personal hygiene. She is pursuing Social Security Disability benefits. Her lawsuit already settled. She has hypothyroidism, controlled with medication, but no other history of significant injuries or illnesses. She has a history of inpatient and outpatient treatment for alcohol dependence 15 years ago. She drank heavily following her divorce 20 years ago but has been free of alcohol for 15 years. She has no other history of mental health treatment.

The psychologist, wanting to understand this woman's complex condition more fully, decides to administer a battery of tests. He wants to assess overall intellectual functioning, psychological functioning, and pain. However, he wants to keep the battery fairly brief, knowing both that the patient probably will be unable to tolerate lengthy testing (because of her reported pain, poor frustration tolerance, and tendency to fatigue quickly) and that the no-fault insurance carrier will likely balk at paying for lengthy and relatively expensive services (compared to psychotherapy sessions) and would probably send the case out for peer review or an IME (independent medical exam), which could result in denial of payment or discontinuation of services. A briefer evaluation would be less likely to trigger such a response from the carrier.

The psychologist administers the Reynolds Intellectual Screening Test (RIST), BDI-FastScreen for Medical Patients (BDI-FastScreen), Beck Anxiety Inventory (BAI), Posttraumatic Stress Disorder Checklist-5 (PCL-5), NEO Five-Factor Inventory (NEO-FFI), and the Short-Form McGill Pain Questionnaire (SF-MPQ).

These measures screen for functioning, traits, and problems in areas of interest to this psychologist. The goal of brevity is accomplished. However, noticeably lacking are measures of symptom and performance validity. Aside from three questions on the NEO-FFI which ask test-takers whether they responded to all of the statements, entered the responses in the correct boxes, and responded accurately and truthfully, this battery does not assess validity. A more appropriate evaluation would have been along these lines: RIST, WAIS-IV Digit Span subtest, Brief Battery of Health Improvement-2 (BBHI-2), SIMS, WMT, and MMPI-2-RF. Although a bit longer, this battery is not overly time-consuming and would provide more clinically useful information in the context of multiple psychometric indicators of symptom and performance validity. Additional measures of personality traits (e.g., NEO-FFI), pain (e.g., SF-MPQ) and other constructs of interest could be added as needed, having considered time restrictions and the demands on the patient. Although a lawsuit as a possible incentive for invalid responding is not relevant in this case, other sources of both primary gain (e.g., attention from healthcare professionals) and secondary gain (e.g., pursuit of disability benefits, drugs) could be impacting the patient's ability or willingness to respond honestly and put forth good effort. Adequate assessment of validity that includes appropriate test selection is needed to understand and address this patient's complex clinical needs.

Conclusions

Rehabilitation patients who have a variety of non-brain-related injuries, illnesses, or disorders often benefit from formal assessment of cognition, emotional state, personality traits, pain, and other factors related to their presenting problems and recovery. There are many reasons why such patients might not approach evaluations or respond in a valid manner. The first step in understanding the constructs of interest in the evaluations is to determine whether the results are valid. Thus, as with disorders of the brain, symptom validity assessment is a necessary part of the evaluation and understanding of patients presenting for psychological services for problems other than disorders of the brain. An evidence-based, multimethod approach to validity assessment is desirable, although additional research is needed with these populations.

6 Lifespan Considerations in Validity Assessment

FOR VARIOUS REASONS, although some clinicians routinely use performance validity tests (PVTs) with young and middle-aged adults, there is sometimes a hesitancy to use these tests with pediatric and elderly patients. Recent national survey data shows that the most common justifications given among neuropsychologists for not using PVTs with children is concern about difficulty interpreting the results, particularly in the context of severe cognitive impairment (Brooks, Ploetz, & Kirkwood, 2016). Although not explicitly stated in the survey, our experience is that this concern is related to a belief that children and older adults will have more difficulty passing these measures than young to middle-aged adults, resulting in false positive classifications for suboptimal performance. Some of the other more common justifications cited in the survey for not administering PVTs to children included time considerations, a belief that exaggeration or feigning is usually obvious in the regular pattern of test scores, and a belief that the yield is usually not worth the financial cost.

Given that older adult patients have a common characteristic with pediatric patients in being at the extreme end of the age distribution, it is likely that some or all of the previously cited justifications against PVT use in children would also be applied to older adults (e.g., difficult to interpret, takes too much time). Likewise, another justification against PVT use with children cited in the aforementioned survey that likely also applies to older adults is a belief that clinical cases rarely exaggerate or malinger, making the use of validity tests unnecessary. For example, some might ask what the purpose would be in administering PVTs to an 11-year-old child with a severe traumatic brain injury (TBI) in which there is no claim for financial compensation by the family. Similarly, some might ask what the purpose would be of administering PVTs to an elderly woman who was taken to the evaluation by her children due to suspicion of dementia, especially when she is denying cognitive complaints. These are examples of lifespan considerations in validity assessment that are the focus of this chapter. Specifically, with regard to pediatric and older adult patients, we discuss (1) why validity assessment is important, (2) common pitfalls to avoid when using PVTs with these age groups, (3) suggested validity assessment methods, and (4) future directions.

Why Validity Assessment Is Important with Pediatric and Older Adult Patients

Recognition of the importance of validity assessment with children has evolved over time. The first modern book on malingering in pediatric populations focused on malingering of psychiatric problems in adolescents in forensic settings (McCann, 1998). Although the first national position paper on validity assessment stated that the use of validity assessment methods is medically necessary as a component of a medically necessary evaluation, there was no specific mention of their use with children or older adult patients (Bush et al., 2005). Similarly, practice guidelines published several years later by the American Academy of Clinical Neuropsychology (AACN) (2007) state, "the assessment of effort and motivation is important in any clinical setting" (p. 221) but make no specific mention of children or older adults.

It was not until a consensus conference statement was published a couple years later by the AACN (Heilbronner et al., 2009) that it was explicitly stated that "Effort measures and embedded validity indicators should be applied to pediatric samples" (p. 15), although no further guidance was provided and no specific mention was made of older adult patients. In 2015, the AACN (Chafetz et al., 2015) went further in commenting on the need for validity assessment in children when noting, "children can and do feign impairment on the examination process" (p. 13) in a position paper about validity assessment in the context of Social Security Administration (SSA) disability evaluations. It was noted that pediatric feigning in a compensation-seeking context frequently occurs at the direction of others (usually parents) and is best termed "malingering by proxy." This is highly relevant to rehabilitation professions, because many pediatric evaluations are performed while a parent or guardian is applying for disability benefits through the SSA on behalf of the child.

In sports concussion evaluations with children (and adults) there is also the issue of intentional poor performance on baseline cognitive evaluations (known as "sandbagging the baseline") to avoid later detection of cognitive decline during retesting in the acute postconcussion phase (Schatz & Glatts, 2013). The study by these authors showed that the addition of a commonly used freestanding PVT, the Medical Symptom Validity Test (MSVT) (Green, 2004a), to embedded measures on a computerized cognitive assessment helped readily detect most participants who tried to sandbag the baseline evaluation.

The realization over time of the importance of validity assessment in children dovetailed with advances in the scientific literature on pediatric validity assessment, summarized in a systematic review by Deright and Carone (2015). By this point, the first book was published that was devoted entirely to the importance of assessing performance validity in children and adolescents (Kirkwood, 2015). Also around this time, the first national survey of pediatric PVT use among neuropsychologists was published and showed that 92% and 88% of North American neuropsychologists administered *at least* one PVT (either freestanding or embedded) and one symptom validity test (SVT), respectively (Brooks et al., 2016). On average, the results showed that children were administered one freestanding PVT, one to two embedded PVTs, and one to two SVTs. The top two justifications provided for using PVTs with children were that independent research justified their utility (76.5%) and that they are necessary to validate other test results (68%). One takeaway message for rehabilitation professionals from the recently published survey data is that validity assessment with children is currently considered mainstream practice during neuropsychological evaluations. Another take-away message is that the use of validity assessment techniques in children should not be limited to concerns about malingering in a forensic/compensation-seeking context. Indeed, survey respondents reported a very high frequency of validity assessment use considering that nearly all of them (97.9%) performed clinical assessments and only 32% performed forensic assessments.

With older adults, malingered dementia can occur, although documented instances in the scientific literature are rare. The most famous case of malingered dementia is that of the elderly mobster, Vincent "The Chin" Gigante, who admitted to feigning dementia and insanity to avoid prosecution (Reid, 2003). There is also the famous case of Dr. William Ayres, the former president of the American Academy of Child and Adolescent Psychiatry, who malingered Alzheimer's-related dementia in an initially successful but later failed attempt to avoid prison as opposed to psychiatric hospitalization for child molestation charges (Huet, 2012).

Although the cases of Gigante and Ayres involved malingered dementia to avoid criminal prosecution, Morgan, Millis, and Mesnik (2009) published a case report of malingered Alzheimer's disease (AD) (which was being treated by a nurse practitioner) in the context of a disability evaluation. Gittleman (1998) published a case of malingered AD in a woman who was in an abusive relationship with a man who coerced her to feign cognitive impairment to obtain long-term disability compensation and to justify her presence at home under his scrutiny. Similarly, a recent case report was published of a 59-year-old woman who had been misdiagnosed with mild cognitive impairment (MCI, a potential precursor to early dementia) for 10 years because poor effort had not been accounted for until PVTs were used during a re-evaluation (Roor, Dandachi-FitzGerald, & Ponds, 2016). In that case, the initial evaluation qualified the patient for disability benefits, which she received, and the re-evaluation was requested to determine whether she would qualify for an extension of disability benefits. A review of the topic of validity assessment in dementia cases noted that malingered dementia can occur in personal injury cases involving toxic exposure, alleged medical malpractice (e.g., poor surgical outcomes), and head injury, although no specific cases were cited (Dean, Victor, Boone, Philpott, & Hess, 2009).

There are many reasons besides malingering why pediatric and older adult patients may put forth suboptimal performance during a cognitive evaluation. One of the more common clinical situations clinicians encounter with both of these patient groups is an oppositional attitude toward the testing procedures. Because both children and older adults come from the ends of the age distribution, it is not uncommon for them to be taken to the evaluation by a family member even though they do not fully understand or agree with the reason for the evaluation. This lack of understanding could be due to very young age, poor/no explanations provided by family or referral resources, significant cognitive impairment, and/or poor insight/defensiveness. Even when an adequate explanation is provided for the reason for the evaluation, it is not uncommon for pediatric and older adult patients to become impatient with the evaluation process. In children, this is commonly due to impulsivity, hyperactivity, and attention/concentration impairment. In older adults, impatience anecdotally appears to be related to a patient's recognition that he/she is having difficulty completing some or all of the tests. The statement, "I don't have time to play these silly games" or a similar statement is one that many clinicians have heard during testing of some older adult patients during midtask difficulty. As a result of these various factors, pediatric and older adult patients do not always feel incentivized to cooperate with the examination procedures, resulting in poor effort on the examination.

Although position statements from national professional organizations have yet to specify that PVTs should be used with older adult patients during dementia evaluations, this view has been put forth in the literature. Specifically, Rienstra et al. (2013) noted that using PVTs as part of the diagnostic process will help to avert false positive diagnoses of early dementia. These authors performed longitudinal research showing a strong positive correlation between hippocampal volume and memory test performance in memory clinic patients but finding that this association was virtually absent when patients failed PVTs. In that study, 11% of 170 consecutively referred patients showed noncredible performance on PVTs, documenting that this is a problem that exists in clinical settings. In a book on ethical practice in geropsychology, Bush, Allen, and Molinari (2017) stated, "failure to systematically consider validity issues simply because of the age of the patient is a form of ageism. Using empirically based measures to help determine the validity of test results is no less important for older adult patients than it is for younger patients" (p. 82). Additionally, Donders and Kirkwood (2013) noted, "It cannot be just assumed that anybody with a diagnosed serious neurological condition, including MCI or dementia, will put forth good effort during neuropsychological evaluations, so accurate assessment of symptom validity remains important" (pp. 402–403). In addition, Miller and Axelrod (2018) asserted, "assessing the validity of obtained cognitive profiles in older adults is just as important as in other patient groups" (p. 27). Thus, it should now be clear that formal assessment of performance and symptom validity with older adult populations is a standard of practice.

Validity assessment with children and older adults should not be limited to concerns about exaggeration of problems because underreporting of symptoms is sometimes an area of concern in both age groups. For children, this is particularly the case when they underreport symptoms after a concussion or some other neurological condition in an attempt to obtain clearance to return back to sports (Echemendia & Cantu, 2003). In older adults, patients with dementia are known to sometimes underreport cognitive symptoms and overestimate their abilities due to defensiveness, denial, and/or poor insight or awareness (Wilson, Sytsma, Barnes, & Boyle, 2016).

Performance Validity Assessment Methods with Older Adults

The PVTs designed for adults can also be used with older adults, but, as with children, it is important to take into consideration variables that can affect performance besides poor effort. Examples of potentially confounding factors include visual acuity (due to common problems such as glaucoma, cataracts, and macular degeneration), manual motor impairments, impulsivity, and anxiety associated with limited familiarity with computer use due to generational factors (for computer-based PVTs). As with children, certain test modifications may be needed to work around these confounds (e.g., operating the mouse for an older adult patient with suspected dementia and/or manual motor impairment).

For older adults, the most salient confounding factor to consider is the possibility that an underlying dementing illness could cause scores to fall below established PVT cutoffs. In the largest study of PVT use with dementia patients (204 nonlitigating patients), Dean et al. (2009) analyzed 18 effort indices derived from 12 tests. The results showed unacceptably low specificity values (30% to 70%) on the vast majority of tests, with the only exceptions being two Digit Span indicators (94% for Vocabulary minus Digit Span and four-digit forward span timed score). The latter is the time to repeat four digits forward (cutoff = > 4 seconds). Specificity for the Test of Memory Malingering (TOMM) (Tombaugh, 1996) was only 63%. The results also showed that specificity values generally decreased as the severity of dementia increased. This occurs because all PVTs, no matter how easy, will always require some basic level of cognitive ability. When clinical conditions are severe enough to impair that basic level of cognitive ability (e.g., advanced dementia, extremely low intellectual functioning), test scores can fall below established cutoffs in some cases. There is some evidence that this effect is magnified with increasing age and lower education (Duff et al., 2011).

The problem of decreased specificity of PVTs in dementia cases can sometimes be mitigated by combining various embedded PVT results. For example, a recent study of patients with early AD ($n = 178$) and amnestic MCI ($n = 365$) found unacceptably high false positive rates (as high as 79% in AD) for three embedded PVTs (Loring et al., 2016). However, when combining a conservative threshold of 6 or less on Reliable Digit Span (RDS) (Greiffenstein, Baker, & Gola, 1994) *and* 9 or less (out of 15) correct on a recognition memory test, false positive classifications were reduced to 5% in AD patients and 1% in patients with MCI.

Due to the potential confound of dementia on PVT performance, clinicians need a way to distinguish between PVT scores that fall below the cutoffs due to poor effort versus dementia (or a similar degree of severe cognitive impairment). One way to make such a determination is to construct PVTs that include ability measures in addition to effort measures and to compare the two types of scores. Three PVTs that include effort and ability measures are the MSVT, Non-Verbal MSVT (NV-MSVT; Green, 2008), and the Word Memory Test (WMT) (Green, 2003). The comparison of effort measures and ability measures on these three tests is known as profile analysis and is easy to compute. Although the name of the profile (e.g., Dementia Profile, Severe Impairment Profile) and the criteria have been modified over the years, the essential aspect has always involved contrasting the average score of the effort subtests with the average score of selected ability subtests. This process is only done with patients who score below the cutoffs on one or more of the effort subtests. If the difference meets or exceeds a specified value (e.g., 20 or more points for the MSVT, 30 or more points for the WMT), the clinical profile is met, provided that the patient has a clinical condition that can reasonably be expected to cause genuine severe cognitive impairment. If the psychometric aspect (i.e., difference score) and clinical aspects of the profile are met, then the results on the test are classified as good effort in the context of genuine severe impairment. If the profile is not met, then the results are classified as suboptimal regardless of the clinical condition, unless there is clinical reason to strongly suspect a false positive (e.g., dementia patient 1 point away from meeting the profile criteria, patient fell asleep during the test, significant distraction in the environment).

Published research using profile analysis began with the MSVT, when it was administered in a memory disorders clinic to 63 patients (average age = 68), some of whom ($n = 11$) had a financial incentive to underperform (applying for disability) (Howe, Anderson, Kaufman, Sachs, & Loring, 2007). The results showed that 27 patients (43%) scored below the MSVT cutoffs. However, when profile analysis was taken into account, the false positive rate was reduced to less than 5%. These findings were extended in a follow-up study by Howe and Loring (2009) with 84 patients from a memory disorders clinic (average age = 72), which showed that application of profile analysis with the MSVT yielded a sensitivity of 55% and a specificity of 91%. This study also described the profile of a group of patients who did not fail one of the effort subtests but who had a 20-point or more difference between the mean of the easy subtests and the mean of the hard subtests. Thus, these patients did not meet criteria for the dementia profile because the effort subtests were passed. This profile was instead referred to as the Expanded Dementia Profile or the General Memory Impairment Profile (GMIP) and showed good sensitivity (84%) to independently diagnosed dementia. Over time, some clinicians began to casually refer to the Dementia Profile as the GMIP, leading many clinicians to believe they are synonymous, but this is actually not the case.

Another study that combined profile analysis on the MSVT and the NV-MSVT for 10 healthy adult volunteers asked to simulate dementia showed 80% sensitivity, and the specificity in 10 institutionalized patients with dementia (average age = 82) was 100% (Singhal, Green, Ashaye, Shankar, & Gill, 2009). In a study of 65 neurological patients (21 of whom had dementia), specificity of the NV-MSVT was 99% when profile analysis was applied (Henry, Merten, Wolf, & Harth, 2010). More recently, application of the profile analysis on the MSVT, NV-MSVT, and WMT with 50 well-educated individuals asked to simulate dementia showed sensitivity values ranging from 54% to 94% and up to 100% when all three tests were used in combination (Armistead-Jehle & Denney, 2015). Longitudinal research has shown that older adult patients presenting with a Dementia Profile on the WMT decline more over two years compared to patients who pass the WMT (Rienstra, Klein Twennaar, & Schmand, 2013). Scoring software for the MSVT, NV-MSVT, and WMT computes a best fit statistical analysis with over 100 various clinical and nonclinical groups, including those with early and advanced dementia. In this way, the use of PVTs that include ability subtests can also be of help diagnostically, which provides further justification for their use.

A promising and quick freestanding PVT that clinicians can use with dementia patients is the Coin-in-the-Hand Test (Kapur, 1994). As implied by the name, the test requires the patient to remember and indicate which of two clenched hands the examiner has placed a coin in after seeing it in the examiner's hand for two seconds and then being asked to count backward from ten. Thus, the test operates according to a two-item forced choice format. This format allows the test to be easily used with patients who have moderate to severe cognitive impairment and allows for the calculation of below chance response levels after 10 trials are administered (half with each hand, randomly distributed). On this test, the patient is provided verbal feedback about the correctness of the response. In the original study on the Coin-in-the-Hand Test, five densely amnestic patients with herpes simplex encephalitis scored 100% correct, whereas two suspected malingerers performed around chance level. The test has subsequently been validated in other studies with larger groups of subjects, all of which showed perfect to near perfect performance in the healthy controls, patients with memory impairments from brain injuries who were recruited from rehabilitation units, and the vast majority of patients with severe memory impairment, whereas the vast majority of suspected malingers had more than one error (Cochrane, Baker, & Meudell, 1998; Hanley, Baker, & Ledson, 1999; Kelly, Baker, van den Broek, Jackson, & Humphries, 2005).

Most recently, the Coin-in-the-Hand Test was administered to 45 hospitalized patients with moderate to severe dementia and no delirium (Schroeder, Peck, Buddin, Heinrichs, & Baade, 2012). The results showed that 73% of the patients had perfect scores on the test, 89% had one or no errors, and no dementia patient made more than four errors. Thus, in dementia evaluations, the authors concluded that older adult patients making 2 to 4 errors may be misrepresenting impairment, 5 to 8 errors should be considered extremely suspect, and 9 to 10 errors represents statistically significant below-chance performance.

Clinicians assessing older adults in rehabilitation settings often use cognitive screening measures or brief batteries (Price & Caplan, 2017). Although most brief measures do not have embedded validity indicators, the Repeatable Battery for the Assessment Neuropsychological Status (RBANS) (Randolph, 1998) is one exception. Two performance validity indicators can be derived from standard administration of the RBANS: the Effort Index (EI) and the Effort Scale (ES). The EI, derived from the Digit Span and List Recognition subtests, was initially developed by Silverberg et al. (2007) in the context of adults with a history of mild TBI

(MTBI). The EI has subsequently undergone some studies with older adults. Hook, Marquine, and Hoelzle (2009), using a sample of nonlitigating older adults (mean age = 74.9; SD = 7.3 years), found that nearly one-third (31%) (*n* = 44) would be deemed to have provided suboptimal performance on the basis of the established criteria. Barker, Horner, and Bachman (2010), studying older adult veterans (mean age = 71.7; SD = 9.3 years), obtained modest sensitivity of 0.64 when specificity was set to 0.85 using the TOMM as an external criterion. These authors concluded that the EI is potentially useful with older adults, particularly when supplemented with other PVTs.

Duff et al. (2011) established base-rates of below-criterion performance for the EI in a large sample of healthy older adults (*n* = 796), long-term care residents (*n* = 229), clinically referred older adults (*n* = 156), research participants with amnestic MCI (*n* = 72), and patients with probable AD (*n* = 126). They found that cognitively intact older adults and those with mild impairments had relatively infrequent rates of below-criterion performance (e.g., 3% for the cognitively intact group). However, increasing severity of cognitive impairment was associated with increasing EI failure rates, with 37% of nursing home residents and 33% of probable AD patients scoring in ranges typically considered consistent with suboptimal performance. They concluded that age, education, and level of cognitive functioning should be considered when interpreting EI results and that significant caution is indicated when interpreting EI scores with older adults suspected of having dementia.

In their comparison of older adults (mean age = 76.4; SD = 10.5) with diagnosed memory impairments with a coached simulator sample of younger adults, Dunham, Shadi, Sofko, Denney, and Calloway (2014) found that the EI demonstrated adequate sensitivity (0.89) but poor specificity (0.41). Thus, overall, these studies with older adults indicate that the EI has adequate sensitivity but widely varying specificity. Overall, the EI has been criticized for having unacceptably high false positive rates when used with patients who have true memory disorders (Novitski, Steele, Karantzoulis, & Randolph, 2012).

In response to the limitations with the EI, the ES was developed to help differentiate between memory impairment and suboptimal performance (Novitski, Steele, Karantzoulis, & Randolph, 2012). Derived from the Digit Span, Delayed Recall (List, Story, and Figure), and List Recognition subtests, Novitski et al. found the ES to have superior classification accuracy compared to the EI in the ability to differentiate patients with a history of MTBI from patients diagnosed with amnestic MCI or probable AD. In a comparison of the ES and EI with older adults, Dunham et al. (2014) found the ES to have higher specificity among those with more severe cognitive impairment, whereas the EI had higher specificity among participants with minimal to mild cognitive impairment. In a comparison of the EI and ES in a mixed neurodegenerative disease, Burton, Enright, O'Connell, Lanting, and Morgan (2015) found very high failure rates on the EI (48%), with considerably lower but still unacceptable failure rates (14%) for the ES. Thus, clinicians are cautioned against using the RBANS validity indices with older adult rehabilitation patients suspected of having genuine advanced memory disorders at this time.

Performance Validity Assessment Methods in Children

In the assessment of young children undergoing rehabilitation, it is important to establish that the child is old enough for valid PVT administration based on published information about the test. Other relevant factors to consider include the child's reading level (for verbally based PVTs), developmental maturity level, presence of visual-motor impairments, and/or presence of genuine severe cognitive impairment. For children and older adults, another important consideration for computer-based PVTs is the presence of impulsivity because of the effect that impulsive mouse-clicking can have on test scores. For computer-based PVT use with children in which reading level, vision, manual motor impairments, and/or impulsivity are potential confounding variables, the examiner may need to use publisher-approved test modifications to administer the test. For example, when such concerns arise, it is an acceptable method of alternative administration on the MSVT and the WMT to operate the mouse based on the patient's oral responses (Carone, 2014; Chafetz & Biondolillo, 2012). In addition, in cases where there is concern about a child's reading ability, it is acceptable to read words aloud from a test that a child cannot read when the stimuli are presented. The latter is particularly important if a child does not have a grade three reading level, either developmentally or because of an acquired injury or illness. This practice is necessary because research with children evaluated for clinical reasons showed that those with less than a third-grade reading level score at a relatively low level on the WMT effort subtests, whereas most children with at least a grade three level passed the WMT effort subtests with adult cutoffs (Green & Flaro, 2003). Other researchers have suggested cautious use of the WMT with children below age 11 based on the performance of patients between ages 6 and 17 (Courtney, Dinkins, Allen, & Kuroski, 2003). Those authors also noted that WMT results were significantly impacted by the child's reading level.

One obvious solution to avoiding the reading confounds with some verbally based PVTs is to administer a visual-spatial PVT. The visual-spatial PVT with the most research support in young children is the TOMM. For example, Constantinou and McCaffrey (2003) demonstrated that 98% of mostly healthy children ages 5 to 12 scored above adult cutoffs on the TOMM. Similar results have also been found with clinically referred patients down to age 6 (Donders, 2005) and age 5 (Kirk et al., 2011). However, research has also shown that TOMM scores below the cutoff should be interpreted cautiously in children with extremely low intellectual functioning, visual-impairment, and/or interictal spike and wave activity due to the possibility of false positive errors (MacAllister, Nakhutina, Bender, Karantzoulis, & Carlson, 2009). Some researchers have explored the use of embedded PVTs with children, but a consistent problem is that these tests tend to suffer from high false positive rates, particularly in younger children and those with severe cognitive impairment, because they are based on tests of ability. For example, Blaskewitz, Merten, and Kathmann (2008) found that 59% of second- to fourth-grade children scored below adult cutoffs on RDS but that none of the freestanding PVTs (e.g., MSVT, TOMM) were failed.

Rather than applying adult-based cutoffs on PVTs to children, some developers of pediatric cognitive tests are beginning to create new embedded validity indicators *during* the test development process. For example, the Child and Adolescent Memory Profile (ChAMP) (Sherman & Brooks, 2015) includes a validity indicator based on significantly below chance performance on four 3-item forced-choice delayed recognition memory tests (verbal and visual-spatial). Use of a significantly below chance threshold was chosen as an indicator to reduce false positives, but the trade-off of such conservative criteria is reduced sensitivity. The test can be used with children down to age 5, was normed on more than 1,200 individuals (representative of the 2012 US population), and no manual motor responses are required. More recently, Sherman and Brooks (2016) published the first pediatric PVT specifically designed for children, which was co-normed with the ChAMP. This test, known as the Memory Validity Profile (MVP), presents the patient with 16 verbal items (half single numbers and half two-letter combinations) and 16 visual-spatial items (half blurred and half heavily blurred colored pictures) followed by a 4-second interval in which the patient is asked to select which of three items was shown. The MVP uses age-adjusted cutoffs (age 5, ages 6 to 10, ages 11 to 15, and ages 16 to 21) to reduce false positive errors across the developmental spectrum. The MVP showed 100% sensitivity and sensitivity to detecting feigned memory impairment during a validation study but is in need of independent validation.

Profile analysis (described in the prior section) on certain freestanding PVTs is another method that can help to reduce false positive rates when PVTs are used with children receiving rehabilitative services. For example, high specificity was found when profile analysis on the MSVT, NV-MSVT, and WMT was applied to children with developmental disabilities (Green, Flaro, Brockhaus, & Montijo, 2013; Harrison, Flaro, & Armstrong, 2015). Larochette and Harrison (2012) showed that profile analysis on the WMT reduced the false positive rate from 10% to less than 1% in children (ages 11 to 14) with severe reading/learning disorders.

Symptom Validity Assessment Methods in Children and the Elderly

With regard to assessing the reliability and validity of symptom reporting, the most common measures used with children are the Minnesota Multiphasic Personality Inventory-Adolescent (MMPI-A) (Butcher et al., 1992), the more recent MMPI-A Restructured Form (MMPI-A-RF) (Archer, Handel, Ben-Porath, & Tellegen, 2016), and the Personality Assessment Inventory-Adolescent (PAI-A) (Morey, 2007). The MMPI-A and MMPI-A-RF can only be used with children down to age 14, whereas the PAI-A can be used with children down to age 12. With regard to overreporting, the PAI-A contains a Negative Impression (NIM) scale to assess the degree to which one endorses items that would present an exaggerated unfavorable impression or that are quite bizarre and unlikely based on comparisons to healthy controls and clinical samples. The PAI-A also contains an Infrequency (INF) scale to assess the degree to which one endorses very low frequency items in comparison to healthy controls and clinical samples, but it differs from the NIM scale in being neutral with respect to psychopathology. High scores on the INF scale suggest a failure to interpret, comprehend, or attend appropriately to item content. The MMPI-A and MMPI-A-RF contain validity scales that assess the consistency of responding (e.g., random or fixed response sets) and the degree of infrequently endorsed items. Symptom validity assessment methods covered in chapter 3 (e.g., other MMPI-2-RF validity scales) could also be used when assessing symptom reporting by older adults.

For assessment of emotional and behavioral functioning in children younger than age 12, the Behavioral Assessment Scale for Children-2 (Reynolds & Kamphaus, 2006) can be administered to children as young as 8 years of age and contains validity indices to help judge the quality of responses. Parent, child, and teacher rating forms are available, which also include validity indices. The validity indices measure the degree of infrequent responses (F index), the consistency of ratings on similar items (Consistency Index), and the presence of an abnormal response pattern (Response Pattern; e.g., cyclical responses, "yes" or "no" response sets). For the assessment of executive functioning complaints, the Behavior Rating Inventory of Executive Functioning-Second Edition (BRIEF-2) (Gioia, Isquith, Guy, & Kenworthy, 2015) can be administered to children beginning at 11 years of age and includes an infrequency scale to help identify unusual responding. An informant version is also available.

Memory problems are a very frequent complaint of patients evaluated in neurorehabilitation settings. As such, it is important to have quicker tools to evaluate the validity of reported memory symptoms than would be afforded by lengthy omnibus personality tests. One option is the 58-item, Memory Complaints Inventory (MCI) (Green, 2004b), which was normed on adults and can be used with geriatric patients. However, clinical judgment is needed to determine whether the test is appropriate to administer to certain geriatric patients (because it is computerized) or whether the test needs to be modified (i.e., reading the items to the patient). Although clinical experience indicates that the MCI can be used with children down to age 12 with a least a grade four reading level (consistent with some other pediatric self-report scales), there are no published studies on using the MCI with children or adolescents, and use of the test with children is considered experimental.

One solution to the experimental nature of the MCI with children is the newly published Multidimensional Everyday Memory Ratings for Youth (MEMRY) (Sherman & Brooks, 2017). MEMRY is the first nationally standardized rating scale for children (self-report down to age 9) for the assessment of memory, learning, and executive aspects of memory (e.g., working memory). There are also parent and teacher versions. Importantly, the measure also contains validity scales to detect inconsistent responses across pairs of similar items (Inconsistency Scale), excessively negative responses (Maximizing Scale; the degree to which items were endorsed as *almost always* which were least likely to be endorsed this way in the standardization sample), or implausible responses (Implausibility Scale; symptoms that almost never occurred in clinical practice, even in patients with severe impairment). The MEMRY authors established the psychometric validity of the validity indicator cut scores by utilizing data from simulation samples (youth and parents) instructed to feign symptoms.

With regard to underreporting, the PAI-A contains a Positive Impression (PIM) scale to assess one's tendency to deny common shortcomings that most individuals would readily acknowledge. The MMPI-A and MMPI-A-RF each contain similar measures of underreporting via the L/L-r and K/K-r scales, respectively. The former is a measure of rarely claimed moral attributes or activities, whereas the latter is a measure of uncommonly high reported levels of adjustment. The level of T-score elevation on the overreporting and underreporting scales from the PAI-A, MMPI-A, and MMPI-A-RF reflects whether the clinical scales (measuring physical, cognitive, and emotional/personality symptoms) can be interpreted, can be interpreted with caution, or are uninterpretable.

Although some patients with dementia are clearly too cognitively impaired to reliably complete a lengthy personality inventory, Carone and Ben-Porath (2014) published a case report of a 65-year-old woman with dementia who was able to reliably complete the MMPI-2-RF despite severe memory impairments and executive dysfunction. The authors concluded that it was safe to attempt administration of the MMPI-2-RF with dementia patients provided that language, comprehension, and attention/concentration are reasonably intact, that Full Scale IQ is at least average, and that the patient appears sufficiently motivated and behaviorally constrained (i.e., not impulsive or sensation seeking).

Although not direct measures of underreporting or overreporting per se, there are some measures that can be used with children and older adults to assess how well their symptom reporting compares to that of an adult informant on the same set of items. For children down to age 12 and adults up to age 99, the NEO-Five-Factor Inventory-3 wealth of information about effort level (NEO-FFI-3) (Costa & McCrae, 2010) allows for a direct comparison of emotional and cognitive symptom ratings between patients and informants. For adults up to age 99, the Frontal Systems Behavioral Scale (FrSBe) (Grace & Malloy, 2001) allows for a direct comparison of apathy, disinhibition, and executive dysfunction symptom ratings between patients and informants. The more reliable the clinician determines the informant to be, the more likely that significantly discrepant ratings reflect underreporting or overreporting of the patient.

There are numerous qualitative behavioral observations that can be used in conjunction with quantitative validity assessment methods to assess the credibility of a child's clinical presentation. These qualitative methods include but are not limited to signs of passive negativity/aggressiveness (e.g., repeated sighing, eye rolling), active negativity/aggressiveness (e.g., negative comments about the evaluation), repeated signs of a desire to leave, signs of separation anxiety, and general signs of poor engagement with testing (e.g., quick "I don't know" answers). In addition, review of school records (e.g., report cards, prior testing, individualized education plans) often provide a wealth of information about effort level in school, and a review of medical records sometimes provides information about effort and compliance that can be useful for the examiner to consider. See Carone (2015) for a more detailed discussion of the methods described in this paragraph. Although these techniques were originally described in terms of their helpfulness in assessing the credibility of presentations in children, some of these techniques can also be applied to geriatric patients.

Summary and Conclusions

The assessment of symptom and performance validity in children is currently commonplace in pediatric neuropsychological evaluations. Although pediatric validity assessment is still in a stage of relative infancy, clinicians currently have numerous quantitative and qualitative options at their disposal to make determinations about symptom and performance validity in children. Validity assessment research with older adult patients is also considered a standard of practice at this point. Studies with dementia populations have yielded several tests that have high specificity, making it possible to distinguish between suboptimal performance and dementia. However, there are numerous caveats that clinicians must be aware of when using PVTs with children and older adults to prevent false positive identification of suboptimal performance. This caution is particularly important in dementia evaluations, where incorrect identification of suboptimal performance could result in delayed treatment of a genuine dementing illness. Conversely, patients can be incorrectly diagnosed with early-stage dementia when providing poor effort if PVTs are not used to identify noncredible performance.

There is clearly a need for more research on PVT use with children and older adults to further refine validity assessment techniques with these groups. For example, there is a need for more quick and freestanding PVTs for use with children and older adults that are easy to administer, such as the Coin-in-the-Hand Test. In fact, the Coin-in-the-Hand Test would be a good PVT for researchers to norm on young children, given that the test would have an intuitive appeal to children who tend to enjoy figuring out where a hidden object is located. It will also be important for future PVT developers to incorporate ability subtests with freestanding PVTs so that a profile analysis can be performed to help distinguish between genuine severe cognitive impairment (especially for dementia evaluations) and suboptimal performance. There is also a need for more research on embedded effort indicators for children and older adults, particularly due to the brevity of many dementia evaluations that stem from limited patient tolerance capabilities. However, developing individual embedded PVTs with adequate specificity will likely remain quite challenging with these groups because they are based on ability measures. For this reason, sole reliance on individual embedded performance validity indicators with children and older adults is discouraged. Rather, freestanding PVTs should also be used; if embedded measures are used, they typically should be used in combination with other measures based on data from published research (e.g., Loring et al., 2016). Lastly, given the complexity of validity assessment with children and older adults, there is also a need for practice guidelines from national psychology organizations regarding the proper use of PVTs with these groups.

7 Interfacing with Rehabilitation Colleagues about Validity Assessment

VALIDITY ASSESSMENT IS a broad topic with many complex components as described throughout this book. Patients and treatment teams benefit when healthcare providers in rehabilitation settings who are knowledgeable about validity assessment understand how to interact with other healthcare providers who are not as familiar with the topic, and vice versa. There are sometimes instances when one healthcare provider is the *only* individual on the rehabilitation team familiar with validity assessment. Typically, this healthcare provider is a psychologist, but it can also be another professional.

Different education and training backgrounds in validity assessment combined with differing assessment and treatment paradigms can pose a significant challenge for rehabilitation team members when communicating about validity assessment. For example, a healthcare provider who interprets patient performance and self-report in the context of objective validity assessment results may experience conflict with a rehabilitation team member(s) who was trained to accept patient performance and self-report at face value. In such situations, when a patient fails validity testing, differing case conceptualizations often emerge, each of which can be met with resistance by the other team member. For example, in an outpatient rehabilitation setting, Roth and Spencer (2013) published a case report in which multiple medical specialists routinely referred a patient with a history of mild traumatic brain injury for neuropsychological evaluations and continued to list brain injury as an active medical problem despite failure on multiple validity tests and conclusions from repeated evaluations that the patient's problems were due to motivational and psychiatric problems rather than brain disturbance. Situations such as these can ultimately result in significant dysfunction within the team dynamic if proactive and ongoing attempts are not taken to address the topic.

In this chapter, we present several mechanisms to facilitate discussions about validity assessment in a productive and interdisciplinary manner. We also discuss ways that healthcare providers with different levels of experience with validity assessment should and should not interact with each other. Lastly, we also cover how to discuss validity assessment with hospital administration officials, who may be brought into discussions about the topic for various reasons (e.g., low patient satisfaction scores, patient complaints).

Didactics

One of the best ways to begin to facilitate discussions about validity assessment on a rehabilitation unit is to schedule an in-service, or series of in-services, about the topic to staff. This can begin with an introduction to the topic followed-up with more in-depth presentations on specific issues over time. Opportunities for audience participation should be encouraged with specific time allotted for questions and discussion. If possible, copresentations with members of different rehabilitation disciplines (e.g., psychology and physical therapy) would be an ideal way to demonstrate interdisciplinary cooperation and agreement on this topic. Case examples from the rehabilitation unit in the context of a broader in-service about validity assessment can be particularly effective at teaching important concepts, especially if the patient is well known to the treatment team.

Case discussions in an open-forum format can also help build team alignment for managing particularly challenging patients. The reason for this is because the nature of the in-person interaction of team members can help facilitate a collaborative exchange of ideas that is lacking when individual team members remain isolated from one other and provide very different case conceptualizations, diagnostic impressions, and treatment approaches via progress notes or clinical reports. This more isolated approach can lead to feelings of defensiveness when one healthcare provider reads in another team member's progress note or report that the team member has disagreed with the manner in which the case was conceptualized or approached. This, in turn, can lead to passive-aggressive behavior among rehabilitation team members and significant team dysfunction. While groupthink should never be the desired outcome of a rehabilitation team, in-person group discussions can at least lead to an open exchange of perspectives so that a common understanding emerges as to why some differences may respectfully exist.

Another helpful didactics approach is to hold a monthly journal club series in which team members from various disciplines are invited to take turns presenting on a peer-reviewed journal article about validity assessment. This is an excellent way to facilitate team building and sharing of ideas and interdisciplinary approaches to validity assessment. The chosen article should be distributed to team members at least one week in advance, followed by a presentation by the speaker on the meeting date. Although one purpose of such meetings is to share approaches and developments on the topic of validity assessment, another purpose is to critique the article for limitations and to discuss areas in need of future research. It is important for presenters to realize that a critique of the article is not a critique of the presenter and that an open discussion is important to better understand the pros and cons of the published research.

An interdisciplinary case conference focused on validity assessment is another excellent way for rehabilitation professionals to come together to discuss cases where validity concerns are present. The format follows the traditional model of other medical case conferences (or "grand rounds") series in which a patient's case history is presented in deidentified format followed by a discussion of examination results, including validity test findings. However, to protect test security, caution should be applied in such settings to avoid presenting validity test stimuli and cutoff scores. For the same reasons, handouts with such information on them should also be avoided. A case conference series about validity should end with an open discussion about the results, the hypothesized reasons for the results, and case management options.

Some rehabilitation team members may also prefer a more personalized approach, which involves a one-on-one meeting for an hour or more to provide a basic overview about validity assessment. This can be particularly helpful for physiatrists, for example, who may be unfamiliar with the psychological tests used for validity assessment that they may see mentioned in reports, whether they are performance validity tests (PVTs) or symptom validity tests (SVTs). Such meetings also provide the opportunity to answer questions that a healthcare provider may not feel comfortable asking in a broader group format.

When providing didactic information to other healthcare providers about validity assessment, it is critical for the presenter to make the point that information learned about validity assessment should *never* be used to coach patients. Coaching about validity assessment techniques is a problem that some healthcare providers need to be mindful of, particularly when there are medicolegal issues involved in the case. For example, Youngjohn (1995) described a case of an attorney who admitted providing an examinee with an article authored by the examiner describing the nature of one of the validity tests that was used during the examination. In that case, the examinee (who had a history of mild head injury at the most) had several areas of impaired neuropsychological test performance that were inconsistent with the neurological history, performed poorly on the validity test he was not warned about, and performed perfectly on the validity test that he was warned about. The author concluded that coaching helped the examinee avoid detection of malingering on the test he was warned about. Wetter and Corrigan (1995) published survey data showing that up to 67% of attorneys felt that they should provide clients with information about validity assessment. Of the 67% of attorneys surveyed, 48% responded that they should always or usually provide this information and 42% stated that they should provide as much information as possible. Given the increased use of validity assessment techniques since the time that survey was published, it would be reasonable to assume that the percentage of attorneys coaching clients about validity assessment has increased over time.

As an example of how coaching can occur in a clinical setting, prior to a patient undergoing a cognitive evaluation with a psychologist, a patient may be told by another rehabilitation team member, "Dr. X is going to give you some tests that measure how much you are trying. Any time he/she gives you a test where you have two choices to pick from, you need to do really well." Alternatively, or additionally, the rehabilitation team member could provide the patient literature on the nature of the tests that will be used, such as an article or a copy of test stimuli. Such actions undermine the assessment process and invalidate the results. For this reason, healthcare providers should take great care not to provide copies of test stimuli during didactic lectures or other educational interactions. If coaching is suspected, there are other options to detect poor effort and malingering (e.g., pattern of performance indices; Suhr & Gunstad, 2000), but it is best to discourage coaching as much as possible.

Motivation for coaching patients about validity assessment or attempting to prevent the administration of validity tests sometimes stems from a misguided attempt to prevent a loss of disability or compensation benefits to patients if the validity tests are failed. A real case example follows. A 54-year-old woman involved in litigation and a workers' compensation claim for prolonged symptoms (13 months at the time) after a concussion from a motor vehicle accident was referred by a rehabilitation psychologist for a neuropsychological evaluation. The rehabilitation psychologist requested during a team meeting that validity tests not be administered during the assessment. The reason provided was that if the patient failed validity tests that this would look bad for her legal case and may negatively impact her future compensation. This request was referred to by the rehabilitation psychologist as an attempt to "prevent harm" even though a discontinuation of benefits would be a reasonable (and just) outcome if the patient did not have a legitimate need for them, and it would free up rehabilitation providers for other patients who do have a legitimate need for their services. There can also be financial motivations for the rehabilitation clinic to prevent the administration of validity tests such as an attempt to avoid the decreased revenue that would occur if the insurance company refuses to pay for continued treatment based on invalid test results and/or evidence of malingering. We know of one instance where this occurred in a rehabilitation chronic pain clinic.

The neuropsychologist explained to the rehabilitation psychologist that a request to omit validity tests violates the standard of care of a neuropsychological evaluation and that it is the responsibility of the evaluator to determine whether the results are valid. The rehabilitation psychologist rescinded the referral and administered a small battery of cognitive tests to the patient while omitting validity tests. Almost all of the scores on the examination were at or below the first percentile (which in and of itself would not be a valid finding in the case of concussion), and the data were interpreted as reflecting cognitive impairment due to concussion, even though there was no scientific basis to make such an interpretation. Additional ongoing rehabilitation treatment was suggested. Afterward, a psychologist hired by the patient's insurance company to review the patient's file to determine whether the prolonged rehabilitation treatment (e.g., occupational and physical therapy, "brain injury" education and supportive counseling by the rehabilitation psychologist) was still medically necessary contacted the rehabilitation psychologist and informed him that his interpretation of the cognitive test results would not be considered because validity tests were not administered. The rehabilitation psychologist was then told to refer the patient for a neuropsychological evaluation in which validity tests were used. The patient was the re-referred for a neuropsychological evaluation. She performed very poorly on most of the exam while egregiously failing all validity tests, most likely due to malingering. It is unknown what happened with her case afterward, as the neuropsychologist's role ended after completing the evaluation.

While it is problematic to try to coach patients about validity assessment results or prevent them from being administered, it is equally problematic for rehabilitation healthcare providers to ignore evidence of validity assessment failure. To this point, Carone (2014) published a case study of a patient who was found to be exaggerating and/or malingering 1 year after an alleged concussion due to a fall at work. The patient was evaluated by a neuropsychologist upon the referral of a physiatrist in the context of a workers' compensation claim, attorney involvement, and possible civil litigation. The concussion diagnosis, extensive and expensive protracted rehabilitation treatments, and disability form signatures by multiple rehabilitation healthcare providers were based primarily on self-report and in some cases behavioral observations (e.g., crying) but not on objective data. After the physiatrist received the neuropsychological test report, she was contacted by the patient via telephone to request that her disability rating be increased from 50% to 100%. If not, the patient informed the physiatrist, the workers' compensation court judge stated that her benefits would be discontinued. Medical records revealed that, based purely on this phone call, the disability rating was quickly increased to 100% and a written statement was made that the patient's complaints were consistent her injury, even though it was blatantly clear that this was not true. No physical exam was completed, and no objective tests were administered to support a 50% increase in disability status. Moreover, the existing neuropsychological testing results showing unequivocal evidence of invalid data were completely ignored. The patient's disability benefits were continued, and she received years of follow-up rehabilitation "treatment" while her case continued to progress through the workers' compensation and legal system. The motivation behind the actions of the physiatrist in this case was likely a desire to avoid confrontation with the patient and to avoid dealing with extensive patient complaints, which the patient had a documented history of filing against other healthcare providers over the years who did not accede to her demands.

As Carone noted in the aforementioned article, while patient advocacy can be an appropriate function for psychologists and other rehabilitation healthcare providers, there is no ethical obligation to automatically align with a patient to facilitate a patient's (or family member's) preferred legal outcome, disability outcome, diagnostic label, medication request, or other such preference. In addition, data should not be suppressed, subverted, or ignored that would lead to increased clarity as to whether such requests are appropriate. The proper basis for patient advocacy is established by using objective scientific methods, including those that establish whether the examination results are valid. In this way, clinical judgment for diagnostic decision-making, treatment planning, and case management is not precluded but supplemented.

Case Discussions

Reaching out to individual team members (or multiple team members separately or together) is an excellent interdisciplinary mechanism to gather and share concerns regarding validity assessment before and after a patient is evaluated. Use of this approach sometimes begins by familiarizing oneself with the referral in advance through a cursory review of records or information communicated about the patient by another team member or the person scheduling the appointment. The healthcare provider may observe, for example, that the patient has been frequently attending physical therapy and occupational therapy sessions. The healthcare provider may also see some information in the medical record that raises concern about patient cooperation or validity. This can include frequent no-shows, noncompliance with homework assignments, extremely high ratings on self-report symptom scales or pain rating scales, unusual behavioral observations, and so forth. A conversation about such a patient can begin with a simple statement such as, "I saw that Mr. Smith is on my schedule and that he has been coming for treatment with you. Have there been any concerns about his effort or the validity of his presentation during those sessions?" This question can be asked without providing background information about reasons for suspected validity problems, or the healthcare provider may choose to provide additional information about why this question is being asked. These conversations can occur in private, in an outpatient group rounds setting, or in an inpatient rehabilitation team meeting.

In some situations, the healthcare provider may not have the opportunity or a clear reason to ask another rehabilitation professional about any validity concerns before the patient is evaluated. In such situations, the healthcare provider may choose to approach another rehabilitation professional if concerns emerge about validity during the initial patient encounter. An example follows. A middle-aged, highly educated patient arrives for an outpatient cognitive evaluation in the context of an open disability claim due to alleged cognitive and motor symptoms after a concussion sustained 1 year prior. During the evaluation, the examiner notices some unusual behaviors on the part of the patient during a mental status and neurobehavioral examination such as inconsistent grip strength, inconsistent visual field problems, and unusual command following. These types of inconsistent presentations typically occur in patients who are exaggerating and/or feigning their presentation because it is difficult to remember and closely replicate how one performed in the past, especially over multiple evaluations spread over longer periods of time. Variable effort over time due to other reasons (e.g., significantly variable fatigue levels, depression levels, pain levels, or general motivation) can also lead to significant inconsistencies in presentations over time, which is why it is important to try to account for such factors during serial assessments. Returning to the case example, after the session and before further testing is completed, the examiner approaches the patient's physical therapist to ask if any inconsistencies have been noted in the patient's presentation. One reason to ask this question, even if there is no mention of inconsistencies in the progress note, is because healthcare providers sometimes refrain from including such inconsistencies or suspicions of exaggeration in the progress note to avoid problematic interactions with the patient.

In the scenario just described, the physical therapist could genuinely respond that no concerning behaviors regarding validity were observed or that some concerning behaviors regarding validity were observed. Such conversations can be very productive because they can lead to the physical therapist (or other healthcare provider) becoming more alert to potential exaggeration in future patient interactions. The discussion may also lead to a decision to administer similar tests (e.g., hand dynamometer grip strength testing, speeded peg placement) in multiple environments to explore whether the patient is responding in a valid manner in one setting but not another. If so, this would naturally lead to some consideration as to why an inconsistent presentation across settings might be the case. If the physical therapist responded that validity concerns were observed in physical therapy sessions, exchange of information about this would lead to convergence of findings across settings and reinforce validity concerns that may not otherwise have been known.

The worst-case scenario in such an interaction would be if one healthcare provider withheld concerns about validity concerns from the other or became defensive about being questioned. An example would be if the physical therapist responded that the patient has always responded in a consistent manner from the beginning of treatment to the present and that no validity concerns were ever observed. Afterward, the healthcare provider who raised concerns to the physical therapist performs a comprehensive records review and discovers that grip strength has been very inconsistent across sessions, with significantly low right-sided grip strength and high left-sided grip strength during some sessions and vice versa during other sessions. The healthcare provider returns to the physical therapist with this information and is told that this information was known during the initial discussion but withheld due to fear that sharing such information would be harmful to the patient. For interdisciplinary discussions to be productive, it is critical that healthcare providers be open and honest with one another. As was explained by Carone (2015), perceived patient advocacy responsibilities should not improperly supersede the need to be objective, honest, and accurate. While there are proper times to advocate for patients when the data supports it, healthcare providers are not automatically obligated to advocate for a patient's disability requests, desired litigation outcome, academic accommodation requests, diagnostic preference, or medication requests. In fact, one of the main reasons that validity assessment is so important is that it helps determine where such patient requests and preferences are appropriate.

Case discussions about validity failure are particularly important when a patient is determined to be malingering to obtain medications. This is a common problem in society that sometimes emerges in rehabilitation settings as malingering to obtain controlled substances (e.g., opioid analgesics for chronic pain complaints, neurostimulant medications for attention/concentration complaints) for personal abuse or resale. Malingering for medication is sometimes detected based on PVT failure in the context of medical records review of "doctor shopping" for medications, repeated claims of losing medications that are sometimes far-fetched, toxicology results suspicious for abuse, repeated requests for increased doses of the medication over time (i.e., after claiming that the lower doses are not helping to relieve the symptoms), and a dubious physical etiology of the alleged symptom(s).

In some situations, a rehabilitation professional may find him/herself in a situation in which another team member (e.g., a nurse practitioner) is the individual overprescribing medication to a patient who is malingering. In such situations, communication of the findings in a report may not be a sufficient way to address the problem. In addition to raising the issue in the report, we recommend scheduling a meeting with the healthcare provider prescribing the medication in which evidence is presented to support the suspicions or conclusions of malingering for medication. Ideally, if the prescriber agrees, a plan can be developed in which discussion with the patient is planned and the medications are tapered/discontinued over time. If there is disagreement, a mutually agreed on plan can be developed for the rehabilitation provider and prescriber to further monitor and discuss the situation over time.

Research

Interdisciplinary research collaboration is an excellent way to promote exchanges about validity assessment in rehabilitation settings. One example would be when one healthcare discipline helps another explore the prevalence of validity test failure with measures not ordinarily at their disposal. An example is the study by Fleming and Rucas (2015) in which occupational therapists were permitted to use a popular PVT developed by a neuropsychologist. Although the study was performed in a private practice medical-legal setting, it is a useful role model for rehabilitation settings. The study showed a PVT failure rate of 48% in that setting, which highlighted the need for some form of validity assessment among occupational therapists.

Another good example of research collaboration about validity assessment was the study by Armistead-Jehle, Lange, and Green (2016) showing the collaboration of the neuropsychology and physical therapy disciplines. The study showed a high (70.5%) correlation between cognitive effort test failure and poor effort with regard to balance assessment. The finding is important because it shows that if performance is not valid in one domain it is likely to be invalid in other domains, a concept previously demonstrated by Green (2007). Developing a common understanding about this among rehabilitation services is greatly needed. For example, if a physical therapist were told that a patient performed poorly on PVTs during a cognitive evaluation, it would be wrong for the physical therapist to assume that poor effort is not occurring during the physical therapy evaluation.

Types of Interactions to Avoid

In addition to avoiding the withholding of validity concerns about patient performance/responses, there are a few other types of interactions that rehabilitation providers should try to avoid to promote a healthy working environment. One example is asking healthcare providers to not use validity tests due to concern that the results may harm the client. Such requests serve to create a dysfunctional team dynamic because it is a request to supersede a standard of care (in neuropsychological evaluations) and/or a request to interfere with attempts to confirm valid data acquisition. Furthermore, such requests typically wind up backfiring in the long run. An example follows. A patient is referred to a rehabilitation psychologist or neuropsychologist for a cognitive evaluation in the context of an ongoing disability evaluation. The referral source has formed a close bond with the patient and states during a team meeting that he believes it would be best if the psychologist did not administer validity tests because poor validity test results may lead to a disability claim denial. The psychologist refuses to accede to the request and both parties become frustrated. Dysfunction can spread among team members who are colleagues of both healthcare providers. The referral source decides to instead administer cognitive tests to the patient, and numerous extremely low scores are obtained that are incompatible with the clinical history. A report is written and reviewed by the disability insurance company. The insurance company hires a psychologist to review the report, which is discounted because no validity testing was performed. The psychologist from the insurance company instructs the referral source to refer the patient for a psychological evaluation that includes validity testing. The patient is referred back to the original psychologist, who conducts the evaluation, and finds a failure on all validity tests. The conflict caused in this scenario could be avoided entirely by being unobstructive with regard to validity testing and appreciating the useful information it provides.

Another type of interaction to avoid is directly criticizing another rehabilitation healthcare provider in a progress note or report. This includes not criticizing other healthcare providers who failed to detect validity concerns during their interactions with the patient (whether or not such concerns should have been obvious) but also includes not criticizing healthcare providers who report validity test failure. An example of the latter typically includes reinterpreting the report of another healthcare provider, sometimes at the request of the patient, and providing one or more unsubstantiated reasons for why validity testing failure occurred. Such a situation typically occurs when a healthcare provider is highly invested in a particular case conceptualization (e.g., that the patient's symptoms are all due to brain injury, that the patient is 100% totally and permanently disabled). A better approach in addressing situations where there may be a disagreement is for rehabilitation team members to discuss why they view the matter differently and to not allow close personal/professional relationships between team members to preclude such a discussion. The written report should ultimately reflect the objective findings of the examination without any personal animus directed to another healthcare provider's conclusions. Differing opinions will be self-evident to a reader of the medical records without the need for one healthcare provider to criticize another in the report.

Healthcare providers should also not ignore the conclusions of another in their reports or progress notes, even if there is disagreement. For example, although one healthcare provider may disagree with another healthcare provider's conclusion that a patient has "postconcussion syndrome" or is totally and permanently disabled, it is best to acknowledge the conclusions of healthcare providers in a medical records review so there can be a complete accounting of the history. In addition, while a healthcare provider may not be pleased to hear about the results of certain testing (e.g., failed validity testing; long-term video EEG monitoring showing psychogenic nonepileptic seizures), it is best to acknowledge this in the progress notes or reports, especially if the healthcare provider is the one who ordered the tests. Failure to do so makes it appear as though an attempt is being made to hide certain results and can cause discontent if a healthcare provider feels that his/her evaluation results are being ignored.

Interfacing with Hospital Administration

In addition to interfacing with other healthcare disciplines, it is important for those working in hospital or other institutional settings to educate the administration about the importance of validity assessment and reasons why validity testing failure can occur. This is particularly important due to the growing emphasis on patient satisfaction scores in hospitals across the country, which links financial incentives to these scores. Specifically, hospitals are financially rewarded or penalized based on patient satisfaction scores as part of the Affordable Care Act. To obtain financial rewards (which can amount to millions of dollars depending on patient volume) many hospitals have implemented a "patient first" culture, patient experience departments, and chief experience officers. While there are certainly many good reasons to measure patient satisfaction, there are instances in which proper medical care and conclusions run counter to a patient's satisfaction. Examples include patients who are refused requested antibiotics because the evidence indicates that they actually have a viral infection, patients refused opiate analgesics due to concerns of substance abuse, patients not provided a disability note when requested, and patients who do not receive a diagnosis of a cognitive disorder due to invalid test data and/or malingering. If healthcare providers believe that they will be penalized for low patient satisfaction scores, the end result will likely be acceding to patient requests for unnecessary care and unreasonable requests (Mehta, 2015).

It is important for healthcare administrators to understand that high patient satisfaction does not always equate to high-quality care. For example, one study showed that patients with higher patient satisfaction scores used more healthcare resources in general, more prescription drug expenditures, and were more likely to die (Fenton, Jerant, Bertakis, & Franks, 2012). As those authors noted, "Without additional measures to ensure that care is evidence based and patient centered, an overemphasis on patient satisfaction could have unintended adverse effects of healthcare utilization, expenditures, and outcomes" (p. 410). Interestingly, research has also shown that patients who put forth poor effort on neuropsychological testing use more healthcare resources, creating an unnecessary resource burden and costs (Horner, VanKirk, Dismuke, Turner, & Muzzy, 2014). Those authors noted that invalid test results may serve as a marker for a more general lack of cooperation with their own healthcare (e.g., not adhering to treatment suggestions) which can then result in further use of healthcare resources. These results suggest that if healthcare providers were more aware of validity problems earlier in the evaluation and management process more cost-efficient care could be provided. Thus, validity assessment should be viewed by healthcare administrators as a helpful and critical aspect of the evaluation and management process and not as one that should be discouraged, even if that means occasionally lower patient satisfaction scores.

Future Directions

A main source of the problem with regard to interdisciplinary communication about validity assessment is that each profession currently differs with respect to the emphasis placed on validity assessment. We believe that future interdisciplinary communication about validity assessment would be significantly improved if more national organizations (e.g., American Physical Therapy Association, American Occupational Therapy Association, American Board of Rehabilitation Psychology, American Board of Physical Medicine and Rehabilitation) representing different professions began to issue position statements regarding the importance of validity assessment. Increased research collaboration about validity assessment between members of different professions will also be helpful in developing a common understanding that can facilitate clinical interactions and communications. Eventually, we envision a time when members of various rehabilitation professions come together in a consensus conference to issue an interdisciplinary statement about the importance of validity assessment and suggested validity assessment approaches in clinical and medicolegal settings.

Summary and Conclusions

Interdisciplinary discussions about validity assessment are important in rehabilitation settings and can be accomplished via various mechanisms such as interactive didactic lectures, case discussions, and research collaboration. Communication about validity assessment in rehabilitation settings needs to be based on an honest and respectful exchange of ideas and empirical evidence to promote an environment of trust and collaboration among healthcare providers. There are several types of interactions to avoid about validity assessment that will help prevent team dysfunction. It is also important for hospital administrators to have a general understanding of validity assessment issues so that they can better understand its value and to help provide context for the occasional patient complaint about conclusions stemming from validity test failure. We are hopeful that in the future more interdisciplinary communication about validity assessment will lead to increased interdisciplinary research on this topic and the first interdisciplinary consensus statement about the importance of validity assessment in clinical and medicolegal settings.

8 Understanding and Managing Invalid Presentations in Rehabilitation Psychology and Settings

ONE OF THE main reasons why validity assessment is often avoided in clinical settings is because of apprehension and concern about how to explain invalid results in reports and how to provide feedback about the results. We believe that this apprehension is primarily due to concern that conveying information about invalid data will threaten rapport and provoke hostile responses, confrontational encounters, and complaints because such a message may imply that the patient is faking or purposely exaggerating. This is a particular concern in rehabilitation settings, where strong bonds and trust are often formed between the healthcare provider and patient (including the family) to facilitate investment in continuing therapy, enhancing behavioral change, and improving treatment outcomes (Danzl, Etter, Andreatta, & Kitzman, 2012; Garberding, 2009; Harman, Macrae, Vallis, & Bassett, 2014). The strong relationships that develop in rehabilitation settings often lead to a strong tendency for healthcare providers to advocate for and protect their patients.

Conflicts often emerge in rehabilitation settings between perceived patient advocacy responsibilities and the need for objectivity, accuracy, and honesty (Carone, 2015). When the former is given priority over the latter, it can lead to unnecessary or misguided testing and treatment. To prevent this from happening, rehabilitation professionals are advised to first establish the validity of a patient's presentation and then to advocate as appropriate. In this way, clinical judgment is not precluded but is supplemented with objective data (Guilmette, 2013). For rehabilitation professionals

Understanding Invalid Presentations

to feel more comfortable achieving this balance, understanding the causes of invalid presentations and how to manage them is important.

Understanding Invalid Presentations

Invalid presentations take on many forms, including but not limited to malingering. In this section, we discuss various reasons for invalid presentations and offer suggestions for avoiding noncredible explanations of noncredible test results.

MALINGERING

Malingering is the intentional production of false or grossly exaggerated physical or psychological symptoms motivated by external incentives (American Psychiatric Association, 2013). A common misconception is that the external incentives that motivate malingering are restricted to financial gain (e.g., disability payments, workers compensation payments, personal injury lawsuits). In actuality, external incentives in malingering also include obtaining drugs (e.g., neurostimulants and opioids), obtaining academic accommodations, avoidance of criminal responsibility, and/or avoidance of responsibility such as work, military duty, and household duties. In an outpatient rehabilitation setting, several cases were presented of noncredible effort in children during a neuropsychological exam in the context of unexplained academic decline (Kirkwood, Kirk, Blaha, & Wilson, 2010). In some of these cases, the authors concluded that validity failure was due to avoidance of responsibility (e.g., schoolwork, playing quarterback) and secondary gain (an attempt for more educational assistance) and could hence be described as malingering. Thus, it is crucial for all rehabilitation professionals to understand the social context of the evaluation because it can potentially explain atypical clinical presentations. Likewise, if it has been established that such external incentives are not present, the clinician would need to consider alternative explanations for validity test failure.

Another common misconception about malingering is that it only applies to individuals who are completely fabricating their entire clinical presentation. Therefore, the reasoning goes, if the patient appears to be reporting some genuine symptoms or has some genuine functional deficits, malingering is impossible. Such a view is overly simplistic and only accounts for what Resnick (1997) described as *pure malingering*. However, as Resnick (1997) pointed out, there are other forms of malingering such as partial malingering (exaggerating actual symptoms or reporting past symptoms as if they are continuing) and false imputation (deliberate misattribution of actual symptoms to the compensable event). Thus, individuals can experience legitimate symptoms and have serious medical diagnoses (e.g., severe traumatic brain injury) and still be malingering.

Definite malingering of neuropsychological dysfunction is concluded when a substantial external incentive is present, if one or more very strong indicators of exaggeration/fabrication of symptoms are present, and if behavior meeting this criteria are not substantially accounted for by psychiatric, neurological, or developmental factors (Slick & Sherman, 2013; Slick, Sherman, & Iverson, 1999). Very strong indicators of malingering include significantly below chance performance on a forced-choice performance validity test (PVT), high probability that performance is substantially below ability level on one or more well-validated psychometric indices (i.e., from any well-validated psychological ability test), and self-reported symptoms that are unambiguously incompatible with or directly contradicted by observed behavior and/or test performance. In cases where psychiatric, neurological, or developmental factors cannot be ruled out, probabilistic language can be used, such as probable or possible malingering, based on the nature and extent of convergent evidence (Bush, 2005; Slick & Sherman, 2013; Slick, Sherman, & Iverson, 1999).

Rehabilitation professionals also need to consider instances of malingering by proxy in which a vulnerable examinee presents in a noncredible manner based on the influence or control of another individual. Malingering by proxy can occur in children (e.g., under the influence of an adult) or adults due to immaturity, neurodevelopmental disabilities, cognitive disabilities, psychiatric illness, or a perceived inability to escape or avoid substantial coercion. Examples of malingering by proxy in the literature include children (ages 9 and 13) with documented brain-injury after a motor vehicle accident in the context of parental litigation (Lu & Boone, 2002; McCaffrey & Lynch, 2009), children (ages 9 and 11) with reported learning problems whose parents were applying for Social Security Disability benefits on their behalf (Chafetz & Dufrene, 2014; Chafetz & Prentkowski, 2011), children (ages 9 and 13) presenting with severe behavioral disturbances (Cassar, Hales, Longhurst, & Weiss, 1996; Roberts, 1997), and a 13-year-old child feigning upper extremity disuse at the behest of his parents who were pursuing a legal settlement (Stutts, Hickey, & Kasdan, 2003). For a recent review on malingering by proxy, see Amlani, Grewal, and Feldman (2016).

OTHER REASONS FOR INVALID PRESENTATIONS BESIDES MALINGERING

An important starting point for rehabilitation professionals to remember is that while malingering is sometimes an explanation for failure on validity tests, it is not always the reason. This point is made in position papers and consensus papers by national neuropsychological associations (Bush et al., 2005; Chafetz et al., 2015;

Heilbronner, Sweet, Morgan, Larrabee, & Millis, 2009) and in malingering classification systems (Slick & Sherman, 2013; Slick et al., 1999). As such, validity tests should not be referred to as "malingering tests" even though they are very helpful for detecting malingering in the proper clinical *context* (i.e., identifiable external gain). There are numerous reasons why invalid presentations may occur besides malingering, as discussed in what follows.

Factitious Disorder

In factitious disorder, there is intentional falsification of physical or psychological signs or symptoms to assume the sick role, often for attention-seeking purposes. Factitious disorder differs from malingering because the falsification is not done for identifiable external gain. For example, in an outpatient rehabilitation setting, Kirkwood and colleagues (2010) presented the case of a 13-year-old child who was attempting to play the role of a scapegoat to delay parental separation, which could thus be described as a form of factitious disorder. In other words, the child was reporting symptoms in an attempt to change the family dynamics so that the parents continued to live together to focus on her health and recovery.

Rehabilitation professionals should also be aware of factitious disorder imposed on another, in which a person known to the patient manufactures or exaggerates symptoms in the patient (or coerces the patient to manufacture or exaggerate) for the primary gain of assuming the caregiver role. Although factitious disorder can be differentiated from malingering based on context and a well-documented evidence trail (Bass & Halligan, 2014), the two can co-occur in the same patient if there are multiple motivations (i.e., attention seeking and external gain).

The Impact of Significant Physical and/or Psychiatric Problems

In rare instances, a patient may display extreme behaviors during the examination (including during validity assessment) that are consistent with reported symptoms and an established medical diagnosis. One example includes a patient literally falling asleep during validity testing and other parts of the examination due to objectively confirmed severe sleep apnea, narcolepsy, and/or use of sedating medication (e.g., high doses of sedative hypnotics and/or opioids). Another example includes a patient crying due to severe pain, such as severe back pain during prolonged sitting resulting from an established significant lumbar disc protrusion/herniation. Yet another example would include a patient with epilepsy literally experiencing a seizure during validity testing. It is important to emphasize again that these are rare instances and should only be used as an explanation for invalid test data when it is blatantly obvious that the extreme observable physical sign is interfering with the valid acquisition of data. Other concerning behavioral observations, particularly in depressed and anxious patients, would include frequent sighing, eye-rolling, making self-deprecatory comments, and seeming overwhelmed and/or panicked when presented with cognitive tasks (particularly those that are timed, complex, and have a lot of stimuli present). In such instances, negative expectations and beliefs about perceived task difficulty could potentially lead to task disengagement.

In psychotic conditions, observations of a patient actively hallucinating or reporting auditory hallucinations (particularly of the paranoid type) could lead to a noncooperative test-taking approach and contribute to task disengagement during testing. In schizophrenia, significant rates of poor effort have been observed (Gorissen, Sanz, & Schmand, 2005; Stevens et al., 2014), perhaps due to the negative syndrome of schizophrenia, which is characterized by apathy and avolition. In rare instances, some patients may be so clearly apathetic about or oppositional to the examination that they visibly respond in a random and flippant manner sometimes associated with confirmatory verbal commentary (e.g., "I don't care about any of this"). Such an observation can occur in a patient with psychosis, severe depression, or an elderly patient with dementia and impaired understanding about the need for the evaluation.

In patients with psychogenic nonepileptic seizures (PNES), it has been found that a history of abuse, but not financial incentive or the degree of psychopathology, was associated with PVT failure (Williamson, Holsman, Chaytor, Miller, & Drane, 2012). In fact, a history of abuse in PNES patients was associated with double the rate of PVT failure in that study. This could be explained by dissociative tendencies (which is a form of disengagement) and can be viewed as an extension of medically unexplained presentations that are so common in patients with somatic stress disorders (somatoform disorders) (Binder & Campbell, 2004). Delis and Wetter (2007) proposed the term "cogniform disorder" as a type of somatoform disorder in which the individual tends to exhibit excessive cognitive complaints in widespread areas of life, suggesting a conversion-like adoption of the sick role, manifested primarily as cognitive dysfunction. However, the concept never achieved widespread clinical acceptance as there were no further publications on the topic after it was proposed, and it was not included in the fifth edition of the *Diagnostic and Statistical Manual of Mental Disorders* (American Psychiatric Association, 2013).

Patients with somatoform disorders represent a challenge for explaining validity test failure because of a tendency for healthcare providers to invoke "unconscious" thought processes as a reason for invalid results. However, as Merten and Merkelbach (2013) explained, the assumption that unconscious pathological processes cause PVT failure resorts to untestable conjecture and violates the law of parsimony regarding scientific explanations. We agree with those authors that one should avoid explaining away PVT failure by speculative psychological factors "unless there is clear and independent evidence that such factors serve as causative antecedents" (p. 133).

Iatrogenesis and Diagnosis Threat

Iatrogenesis is when treatment or information provided by healthcare providers prolongs/worsens existing physical and/or mental health problems or causes new ones, despite the best of intentions. An example would a patient becoming depressed, angry, and/or anxious because one or more healthcare providers stated that the nature and implications of the presenting/alleged health condition was much worse than it actually was. Further harm can then be caused by prescribing treatments (e.g., medications, prolonged rest) that cause genuine problems (e.g., concentration problems due to medication-induced fatigue, obesity from inactivity) that did not previously exist. These new problems can then become conceptualized by the patient and healthcare provider as being caused by the presenting/alleged condition when they were actually caused by the interventions. Such patients can easily become psychologically enmeshed in the disability role (especially if the healthcare provider is the first to advocate for disability) and may behave in a manner that reflects more disability than is actually the case (or present as disabled when there is no actual disability). Similarly, some patients may perform worse than their true capabilities of (e.g., on cognitive testing) as a result of the healthcare provider calling more attention than is necessary to symptoms, a problem known as diagnosis threat (Suhr & Gunstad, 2002). For an updated review on medical and psychological iatrogenesis, see Carone (2018).

Underreporting

Although not given as much attention as its overreporting counterpart, underreporting is another form of invalid presentation sometimes encountered in rehabilitation settings. There can be serious neurological causes of this such as anosognosia (reduced/lack of awareness of deficits) after severe traumatic brain injury, or psychological explanations such as denial of deficits/symptoms due to a desire to be seen as normal by others, a desire to return to sports or one's military unit, or an unwillingness to admit to psychological problems. Practitioners also must remember that it is not uncommon for a patient to underreport problems in one area (typically emotional problems) and overreport problems in another area (typically cognitive and physical symptoms). When the latter scenario is psychologically based, the reason is typically because patients tend to view cognitive and physical symptoms as problems that others will perceive as beyond their control (e.g., due to alleged brain injury effects) and psychological symptoms as problems that others will perceive as within their control. Moreover, some patients become concerned that acknowledging psychological problems will later be used as an explanation for their cognitive and physical symptoms if a neurological cause is alleged to be the cause in a compensation-seeking context.

AVOIDING NONCREDIBLE EXPLANATIONS

Healthcare providers must be particularly careful to avoid using noncredible explanations for noncredible examination results. Noncredible explanations are those that do not have solid research support, directly contradict published research support, and/or are not supported by behavioral observation. For example, depression, posttraumatic stress disorder, chronic pain, fatigue, headache, unconscious processes, or medication use are generally not credible explanations for validity test failure (Green & Merten, 2013) unless there were extreme observable genuine behaviors present consistent with the patient's history to support such a conclusion. Invalid presentations should not be explained away by purely subjective complaints (e.g., fatigue, sleepiness, pain) that lack an extreme observable behavioral correlate and clearly established medical or psychiatric cause for the observed behavior. Another example of a noncredible explanation of validity failure would be concluding that it was caused by trying too hard (Silver, 2015) or by defense examiner bias for rehabilitation patients evaluated in medicolegal settings. Neither of these explanations have empirical research support. In fact, the evidence actually suggests that validity failure is more common in plaintiff examinations (Greiffenstein, 2009).

Managing Invalid Presentations

Managing invalid presentations is a challenging situation for most healthcare providers. In this section, we discuss feedback and management approaches for various situations regarding invalid presentation, the use of face-saving techniques, and suggestions for how to manage angry and hostile reactions.

FEEDBACK MODEL AND GENERAL APPROACH

We previously published a detailed model on providing feedback to patients with invalid test performance (Carone, Iverson, & Bush, 2010) and expanded on this model with respect to patients reporting persisting symptoms after mild traumatic brain injury (Carone, Bush, & Iverson, 2013). We refer the reader to those works for detailed explanations of this feedback model but provide a brief synopsis here with additional information about how the model can be applied by nonneuropsychologists in rehabilitation settings. The first phase involves building rapport and obtaining informed consent. This is essential because one cannot expect to have a successful feedback session with a patient about news that can be difficult to hear if the patient does not trust that the healthcare provider is trying to be helpful, yet thorough, honest, accurate, and objective. Good rapport can also assist in facilitating future discussions about underlying reasons for poor effort (Mason, Cardell, & Armstrong, 2014). The informed consent process helps to outline the evaluation process as well as the benefits and risks, such as that (1) there may be unexpected findings, (2) the patient may or may not agree with some or all of the findings and interpretations, (3) no conclusions or recommendations can be guaranteed in advance, and (4) there is no guarantee that the results of a clinical evaluation will be of assistance in a compensation-seeking context (or may have no impact or an adverse impact). For physiatrists, nurse practitioners, and rehabilitation therapists who typically have briefer evaluation times than psychologists, we believe that a brief discussion of these issues is important before the evaluation begins because it helps to establish proper expectation and professional boundaries. There should be a signed consent form for documentation purposes that covers this information, and this is the form that should be discussed with the patient. For rehabilitation providers working in hospitals or medical centers, this would be a different form than the general consent to treatment form that patients or their proxies sign at the registration desk.

The second phase of the feedback model involves completing the evaluation and having a preliminary discussion at the end of the testing session with the patient about his/her effort level if performance-related validity problems were noted. The purpose of this is to see how willing the patient is to acknowledge poor or variable effort. While patients are generally not willing to explicitly say that their effort was poor, we have found that patients are more often willing to acknowledge "disengaging" when perceiving tasks as too difficult or irrelevant. This topic can be easily broached with patients when there is behavioral evidence (e.g., seeming frustrated and/or overwhelmed, sighing, making self-deprecating comments). If no such behavioral evidence exists, patients can be asked to rate the difficulty of easy tasks they were asked to complete and explain why they perceived them as difficult, which can help segue into a discussion of task disengagement. Another way to broach the discussion is to ask the patient if he/she easily disengages from tasks in real-life settings that seem difficult and if this could have occurred during the examination. The healthcare provider does not need to agree with the patient's explanation for task disengagement, but obtaining a preliminary acknowledgment can be very useful in broaching a more in-depth discussion on the matter. This discussion framework can be equally applied to effort-related problems in physical and cognitive presentations and is a discussion that can be had by physiatrists, nurse practitioners, and rehabilitation therapists.

Phase three of the feedback model is the actual explicit discussion with the patient about poor effort and/or exaggeration. Before discussing this phase in more detail, it is important to discuss the timing of the feedback. Although psychologists typically hold the feedback session on a separate day after testing is completed over many hours, the situation is different for other rehabilitation professionals, who hold briefer initial sessions where it may take additional time to accumulate validity data. If suspicions emerge regarding invalid data during a consultation with a physician, nurse practitioner, physician assistant, or rehabilitation therapist, additional data should be gathered to confirm that this is the case before a comprehensive treatment plan is implemented, and this information should be shared in an interdisciplinary manner. This is perhaps one of the most important points of this book. That is, it does not make sense to refer a patient for numerous rehabilitation therapy services and diagnostic tests, and to formulate an extensive and/or indefinite treatment plan without first establishing whether the treated problems are valid and without communicating any concerns as a team. As an example, if a physiatrist suspects exaggerated sensorimotor weakness based on inconsistent grip strength during an initial assessment, it does not make sense to refer the patient for physical therapy unless the physiatrist shares the concerns with the therapist and seeks additional input about validity issues (e.g., functional capacity examination). Yet this is precisely what happens in many instances. It would also not make sense for the physical therapist to continue to treat the patient for an extensive (e.g., 20) or indefinite number of sessions, not addressing the obvious issue with performance validity, and not sharing the concerns with other providers on the rehabilitation team, including the neuropsychologist.

During the feedback session, we strongly advocate taking a nonadversarial approach and using a "good-news bad-news" approach. In this approach, the patient is told that the bad news is that he/she has many areas of low test scores or low-appearing areas of functioning. The patient can also be told that in many cases it is concluded that the low scores and/or functions are severe and permanent. The patient is then told that the good news is that this is not the case for him/her and that the evidence shows that the patient is capable of much better test scores and/or functioning. This approach can be used with respect to cognitive functioning and physical functioning. Although the healthcare provider should avoid revealing to the patient the precise way that poor effort was determined, general information can be provided. For example, a patient can be told that the pattern of the sensorimotor examination performance is not consistent with what is found in genuine neurological disease and does not follow known neuroanatomical distributional patterns. This leads into discussion of the obvious conclusion that there must be an alternative explanation for the examination findings, with the possible factors depending on the context of evaluation, behavioral observations, and what is known about the patient's history. Lastly, focus then shifts to identifying ways to address factors that are interfering with valid test result findings (e.g., referral for psychological counseling, treatment of extreme pain/somnolence, settling of compensation-related claims in a personal injury case).

By using this feedback approach, we have found that the vast majority of patients and their families are accepting of the conclusions. We believe that this is due to attempts to establish rapport with patients and make them feel comfortable; making sure that patients do not feel rushed or as if they are inconveniencing the examiner; showing patients that a thorough, comprehensive assessment was performed; keeping feedback focused as much as possible on objective opinions; avoiding inflammatory language (e.g., "quitter" or "faker"); and using the "good news bad news" approach. For patients who are malingering, the "good news bad news" approach to feedback places them in an awkward social-cognitive situation because it would seem strange for someone to be upset to hear that abnormal examination results are not as bad as they seem and that the brain (or other area of the body) is functioning much better than the results would initially appear to indicate. Although our feedback model was based on anecdotal evidence that it was successful in rehabilitation settings, there was no scientific evidence available at the time that a feedback model such as this could lead to positive outcomes. However, such evidence was recently published when using a similar feedback model with children as is described in the next section.

FEEDBACK ISSUES REGARDING CHILDREN: EVIDENCE OF IMPROVED OUTCOMES

In the case of children, a similar approach can be used as the feedback approach outlined earlier, although in some cases the feedback session may occur with only the parent(s) present. Recently, Connery, Peterson, Baker, and Kirkwood (2016) described a feedback approach for these situations used in a large multidisciplinary concussion program in a rehabilitation setting due to the persisting problem of 15% of pediatric concussion patients presenting with noncredible test results. Their model is similar to ours in that it uses a nonaccusatory but direct approach, exploring reasons for noncredible performance with the caregiver, and making recommendations for management. The authors found similarly high levels of caregiver satisfaction and a greater reduction of self-reported symptoms in patients who received feedback after invalid test results compared to patients who received feedback when no validity concerns were present. These results are important for rehabilitation providers because it shows that there is no need to refrain from providing feedback about noncredible presentations and that providing such feedback can actually be helpful. According to the authors, helping people understand the noninjury aspects of the patient's presentation may be beneficial in improving outcomes.

When the healthcare providers believe it is clear that the caregiver(s) have a solid understanding of why the patient provided invalid test data, the child is asked to join the feedback session. At that time, the good news and bad news approach is used based on modified language from our 2010 feedback model, and the child is asked to provide his/her input. Although some children may admit to poor effort during such a discussion, some will become upset and defensive. Connery et al. (2016) advised against a back and forth confrontation with the child about this topic, but recommended that clinicians reiterate the validity assessment findings and discuss the importance of addressing nonneurological factors in treatment. No specific age cutoff was provided by the authors for allowing the child to participate in the feedback session, and we suggest that the decision about whether to include the child in the feedback session be made on a case-by-case basis.

FEEDBACK REGARDING MALINGERING

In some instances, the evidence in clinical settings overwhelmingly supports a conclusion that the patient is malingering. When this happens, clinicians understandably struggle with how to address the situation. As Stutts et al. (2013) aptly noted, "Confrontation is a difficult part in caring for the patient who is malingering" (p. 278) and that a far easier path would be to simply refer the patient for further testing or procedures. In our experience, there have been instances in which healthcare professionals had suspicions about malingering but later revealed (after malingering was detected) that they did not share those concerns with team members (or actively hid such concerns) due to fear of damaging the provider-patient relationship and fear of complaints and angry reactions. Although such risks can never be totally avoided, especially with such a sensitive topic, we agree with Stutts et al. (2003) that confrontation is a necessary first step in resolving the situation. While those authors were referring to confrontation in malingering by proxy cases, we believe that their recommendation holds true in other malingering management situations.

We recognize that the term "confrontation" may initially seem antithetical to the process of rehabilitation. In military settings, which often involve extensive rehabilitation services, Schnellbacher and O'Mara (2016) opined that patient confrontation is countertherapeutic and that it will lead to malingering patients becoming more invested in their symptoms. LeBourgeois (2007) advocated allowing patients to clarify discrepancies in cases of malingering and to avoid confrontation, but it is unclear how such a process can ultimately lead to resolution of the problem, and it would likely lead to yet further denials by the patient (which would ironically be a confrontation). Approaches to addressing malingering with patients that eschew confrontation generally involve providing patients with very vague explanations, such as "Sometimes other issues are at play that can cloud the clinical picture," and that the patient's test results "correlate with exaggeration" (Schnellbacher & O'Mara, 2016, p. 105). The problem with such an approach is that it does not directly disclose the identified problem, which the patient will likely discover when accessing the clinical report in the medical record, ironically leading to anger that the healthcare provider was not being open and honest during the feedback session. It is also extremely difficult to maintain such an approach in the face of persisting questions for clarification from the patient during a feedback session without being deceptive.

There is common everyday precedent in rehabilitation settings for *respectful confrontation* to lead to positive outcomes. For example, rehabilitation therapists frequently confront patients in inpatient settings who do not want to get out of bed to complete 3 hours of daily therapy, often with good result. In addition, rehabilitation psychologists and physiatrists sometimes need to confront patients who have repeatedly not followed through with treatment recommendations (e.g., completing homework from therapy, sleep apnea treatment compliance, attending psychotherapy), which can also yield positive results. Problematic outcomes related to confrontation likely have less to do with the actual confrontation and more to do with the style of the confrontation (e.g., accusations of lying, shaming the patient, expressing strong indignation, all of which should be avoided). As an example, based on successful police interrogation techniques, Knoll and Resnick (2006) suggested stating, "You haven't told me the whole truth" rather than "You have been lying" (p. 643).

With proper bedside manner, confrontation about malingering can be done in a respectful, objective, and truthful manner while also reminding patients that some of the symptoms they report may indeed be valid. For rehabilitation professionals uncomfortable confronting patients alone about this topic (or invalid results in general), such feedback can be conducted in the presence of a psychologist or psychiatrist who has expertise in the matter. This is a form of "supportive confrontation" that is recommended by Bass and Halligan (2017). Dignity-sparing techniques are an important aspect to feedback about malingering (Schnellbacher & O'Mara, 2016). It is important to avoid the use of inflammatory words and phrases such as "the test results show you are faking (or lying)" and to resist patient attempts to get the examiner to use such words (e.g., "So, you are basically saying I am liar, right?") that would form the basis or a future complaint. Rather than using such terminology (either in reports or during feedback), we suggest being factually and scientifically descriptive. For example, one can state the following during a feedback session:

> "The test results show a pattern of performance that is significantly worse than chance. In other words, even if you had never seen the test stimuli at all you should have done much better purely based on guessing. This indicates that there were times that you knew the correct answer but chose the wrong one. When this happens and there is something significant to be gained and/or avoided by appearing more impaired than you are, there is a term for that known as 'malingering,' which I concluded applies to your case."

This wording can be paraphrased for application to different patterns of test failure such as failure on numerous validity tests that were not below chance (e.g., "There were numerous times during the testing when you performed much worse on easy tasks than children with severe traumatic brain injuries. Since you suffered a mild traumatic brain injury, those results do not make sense biologically and indicate that nonbiological factors are causing you to perform worse than you are capable of."). Physiatrists can also apply this model when talking to patients about noncredible physical examination findings (e.g., "There were several findings on the physical examination that are not biologically possible (or plausible)." The latter can be discussed in the literal sense (e.g., the findings are neuroanatomically impossible for anyone) or in a relative sense (e.g., the findings are not possible for the patient given what is known about their condition). Findings from a neuropsychological evaluation can of course be integrated into discussions with patients about malingering.

We are mindful that some healthcare providers explicitly want to avoid using the term "malingering," referring to it in a taboo manner as "the M word." This avoidance is partly due to understandable social discomfort in situations where patient feedback is expected and fear of reprisals. One strategy to use in such a situation is to avoid use of the word "malingering" but still apply the definition in the report and during feedback as described above. For those who are not comfortable with such an approach and who avoid use of the term because they do not believe that it is ever possible to know a patient's intent, the possibility of malingering can still be mentioned when talking about the possible reasons for validity test failure. As one example of phrasing, one can state that the pattern of test findings do not allow for one to rule out that intentional underperformance for secondary gain occurred. Such wording is a better approach than failing to mention an obvious explanation for validity test failure, depending on the context of the case.

Once a discussion about malingering (or the description of malingering) has occurred, it is important to temper ongoing treatment. Specifically, the discussion about this topic should serve as a foundational reason to avoid referring the patient for more unnecessary medical tests and procedures, tapering and/or discontinuing certain medications and prescriptions, and discontinuing rehabilitation therapies. Of course, if evidence emerged of a genuine problem that should be addressed, then this should be appropriately evaluated and treated. Otherwise, the focus should remain on identifying the reasons for deceptive abnormal illness-seeking behavior to help the patient understand how the behaviors are counterproductive and how to achieve goals in a prosocial manner. Although there is no direct evidence of treatment success in malingering, a referral for psychological counseling would make the most sense as a way to achieve such a goal. Relatedly, various forms of psychotherapy have shown some success in the management of somatization (Lamberty, 2008).

FEEDBACK ABOUT FACTITIOUS DISORDER

Management of factitious disorder involves supportive confrontation about the diagnosis, emphasizing the need for help and harm reduction, and a referral for psychological counseling (Bass & Halligan, 2014). This is true for inpatient and outpatient rehabilitation settings. For counseling to succeed, it is important for the patient to accept the diagnosis and the need for treatment. Reich and Gottfried (1983) found that (1) most patients improved after being confronted about factitious disorders, (2) 13 of 41 patients with factitious disorders confessed to causing their disorders, and (3) four patients became asymptomatic. These findings counter commonly held assumptions that confrontation with such patients will not be helpful. On the other hand, Eastwood and Bisson (2008) found no evidence that any treatment approach was superior for factitious disorder, including confrontation versus nonconfrontation, psychotherapy versus nonpsychotherapy, and psychotropic medications versus no psychotropic medication. However, lack of compliance in these patients severely limits conclusions on efficacy (McCullumsmith & Ford, 2011).

USE OF FACE-SAVING TECHNIQUES

In Pankratz's (1979) original article that contains the first use of the term "symptom validity testing" he applied a forced-choice technique for the assessment of deception in two patients with functional sensory disorders. Pankratz also used the technique to rehabilitate these patients by later changing the context of stimulus administration from assessment to "symptom retraining." The purpose of this was to create a situation in which the patient would be less likely to deny the perception of the stimulus cues. This was facilitated by telling the patient that the procedure was designed for retraining residual sensory signals to the brain. In this way, the patient was permitted to retain their incorrect conceptualization of the problem. This technique attempts to elicit change by avoiding confrontation with the patient about the etiology of the symptom so as to avoid emotional reactions. Pankratz reported the success of this procedure in the return of sensory function in one patient with functional right glove anesthesia, but details on the patient's background are lacking. For the one patient described by Pankratz who appeared to be malingering (in our opinion) for the highest disability benefits that anyone on the hospital staff had ever encountered, he reported a return of touch sensation when a neurological basis was provided for the procedure, but he declined staff attempts to help him with a return of function.

Some clinicians use a double-bind approach to manage malingering, which involves telling patients that they should improve with treatment if they have genuine symptoms and then referring them for treatment of the alleged problem (Schnellbacher & O'Mara, 2016). The problem with this approach is it exposes patients to unnecessary treatment (some of which can be harmful, such as medication side effects) while restricting access to treatment for other patients. Furthermore, there is nothing about this approach that prevents patients from claiming that their symptoms did not improve because there must be something special about their case.

A face-saving technique for managing factitious disorder (that can also be applied to malingering) was developed by Eisendrath (1989) based on his experience that confrontation was generally not helpful. This approach involves first telling the patient that there appears to something present causing a great deal of stress, that it is possible that the person is creating symptoms due to stress and a need for help, and referring the patient for a short course of therapy (e.g., relaxation therapy) that in theory would allow the patient to give up the symptoms without losing face. Four case studies of factitious disorder managed with this approach were used as supportive evidence of its efficacy. However, in some cases, Eisendrath (1989) acknowledged that confrontation is sometimes the only option available. While a nonconfrontational approach may be appropriate in some instances, we urge clinicians not to use false explanations and euphemistic language (e.g., behavior was caused by a "cry for help") when the available evidence does not support such a conclusion.

MANAGING MALINGERING BY PROXY

In cases of suspected malingering by proxy, Chafetz and Dufrene (2014) and Amlani et al. (2016) recommended contacting the local Child Protective Agency (CPA) to report the case as a form of abuse. Importantly, healthcare providers are not required to prove the occurrence of malingering by proxy before filing a report just as they are not required to prove other cases of abuse; that would be the job of the CPA workers after they perform a thorough investigation. Many have specifically recommended a team-based approach to managing malingering by proxy (Amlani et al., 2016; Bass & Glaser, 2014; Stutts et al., 2003). This can include the participation of psychiatrists, psychologists, social workers, allied healthcare providers, teachers, and other prior care providers, including those in rehabilitation settings. As Amlani et al. (2016) pointed out, the safety of the child is paramount in such cases, such as tapering or discontinuing unnecessary medications and having a low threshold to refer the case to other entities including law enforcement. They also noted that long-term follow-up in such cases is essential and that further guidelines for the evaluation and management of malingering by proxy are needed.

MANAGING ANGRY AND HOSTILE REACTIONS

While we believe that our feedback approach minimizes the chances of angry and hostile reactions about invalid data, no feedback approach can completely eliminate this risk. As Bass and Halligan (2014) pointed out, some patients will interpret confrontation as humiliating, seek care elsewhere, lodge complaints, and escalate their self-destructive behavior. Some patients may make personal threats or even file lawsuits, although both are rare. Thorough documentation, objective data, a signed informed consent form that explains the risks of the evaluation, collegial support, feedback in the presence of another colleague, setting firm limits, remaining calm, informing building security guards of patients at high risk for hostile reactions, and sitting close to an unencumbered exit from the room are all ways to manage various levels of aggressive reactions. For detailed information on how to handle patient complaints, see Carone et al. (2010).

MANAGING UNDERREPORTING

Underreported and minimized symptoms can be managed by discussing with patients that there are objective indicators from personality tests indicating the presence of underreporting and/or informing patients that there is a significant discrepancy between the denial of certain symptoms and direct behavioral observations. A common example would be pointing out to a patient that while depressive symptoms were denied, affect was observed to be flat, there was poor eye contact, numerous self-deprecatory comments were made, and numerous instances of crying were observed. In such situations, it is best for a frank discussion to ensue about why the patient is underreporting, with the healthcare provider mentioning some of the likely possibilities (e.g., perceived mental health stigma, preference for an external locus of control, cultural factors promoting stoicism, desire to return to sports). The end-result message in such situations should be that the patient is actually doing more harm than good in not acknowledging symptoms that can be treated, which in turn, can help improve functioning. For treatment suggestions regarding anosognosia, we refer the reader to the behavioral management strategies discussed by Prigatano and Morrone-Strupinksy (2010).

FEEDBACK CASE PRESENTATIONS

This section provides three examples of feedback involving invalid case presentations in rehabilitation settings. The first two cases involve patients in whom there is no actual neurological cause of persistent symptom reports despite them being told otherwise. The third case involves feedback to a patient with invalid test results in the context of a genuine long-term neurological condition. While rehabilitation psychologists evaluate other types of patients besides those with known or suspected neurological conditions (e.g., spinal cord injury, orthopedic trauma, burn injuries) we used these cases as examples because they are the most common contexts in which challenging feedback sessions about validity assessment occurs. Themes and lessons from these feedback sessions can be applied to other types of cases, however.

Case 1: Positive Reaction and Outcome to Feedback

Ms. Doe was a 47-year-old woman referred by a physiatrist for a neuropsychological evaluation. The evaluation was performed 1 year after she suffered a concussion at work due to an assault. Despite the mild nature of her injury, Mrs. Doe had become convinced by talking to her healthcare providers that she suffered a "severe traumatic brain injury." Neuroimaging results were negative. She denied pending litigation but had a contentious ongoing workers' compensation claim. She attended a combined total of 64 outpatient occupational therapy and physical therapy sessions in an outpatient rehabilitation setting for vague persisting symptoms. She only attended nine counseling sessions with a rehabilitation psychologist despite her appearing significantly anxious stemming from the assault reactivating memories from a very traumatic prior history of abuse. The rehabilitation psychologist stated that Mrs. Doe was totally and permanently disabled from employment (which involved driving) due to her subjective visual complaints. Her occupational therapist originally disagreed that she was disabled but eventually relented under pressure from the rehabilitation psychologist to support this decision. At the time of the neuropsychological evaluation, Ms. Doe had no income because she exhausted her sick leave and her workers' compensation benefits were being disputed. As a result, she reported that she was close to being evicted from her home.

On neuropsychological testing, Ms. Doe performed poorly and inconsistently on many PVTs such as providing inconsistent responses and performing better on some tasks that are objectively more difficult than others. On symptom validity tests (SVTs), she presented with overreported memory complaints that had a clear psychiatric component to them (i.e., endorsing items rarely reported by neurological groups and mostly endorsed by psychiatric groups). These complaints (e.g., impairment of remote memory) were likely related to her extensive history of abuse and psychological trauma which had not been disclosed (and does not appear to have been inquired about) by any of her healthcare providers over the prior year of rehabilitation treatment. Her trauma history was considered by the neuropsychologist to play a key role in understanding her current case presentation, which explained why she readily endorsed signs and symptoms of panic disorder and posttraumatic stress disorder. She appeared highly anxious and psychosomatic via behavioral observations but grossly underreported psychiatric symptoms on SVTs. She reported moderate depression during interview and on a brief self-report scale.

During the feedback session, the "good news bad news" approach was used. Ms. Doe was informed that the test results reflected what she was minimally capable of doing. She did not dispute these results and requested direction on what to do regarding employment. It was explained to her that there was no neurological reason why she should be permanently disabled from her job, that she appeared to be mentally stuck in a disability role at the time, and that she believed herself to be severely brain damaged when this was not the case. It was explained to her and her other healthcare providers that the treatment focus needed to be reversed so that the focus was much more on decreasing her anxiety and depression with psychological counseling rather than focusing on physical and cognitive symptoms. A discussion of the effort test results was useful in convincing her that she was much more capable than how she was presenting. It was suggested to her treating providers that she be actively divested of the notion that her brain injury was severe and that she be allowed to return to work on a trial basis. The neuropsychologist contacted the physiatrist to discuss allowing her to return to work, and this request was granted. Ms. Doe subsequently returned to work, performed her job well, and even won an award for high performance. She was able to retain her home. She later thanked the neuropsychologist for "freeing me from the box that I felt trapped in."

This case highlights the importance of taking a comprehensive history that includes a review of prior trauma/abuse and integrating this information along with validity assessment results into the case formulation. This case also highlights the perils and drastic impacts that can occur to patients when they are told that they will never be able to return to work based purely on subjectively reported symptoms. The use of validity assessment techniques at the outset of her presentation in the rehabilitation setting would likely have fundamentally changed the nature of her treatment to obtain a more positive earlier outcome. Lastly, this case highlights how feedback about effort test results can be therapeutic and lead to positive patient outcomes.

Case 2: Adverse Reaction and Outcome to Feedback

Mr. X was a 49-year-old man referred by a rehabilitation nurse practitioner and a physiatrist for a neuropsychological evaluation. The evaluation was performed 9 months after he suffered a concussion during a motor vehicle accident. Neuroimaging results were negative. He was suing the driver of the other vehicle and had been held out of work by the nurse practitioner. With a few additional disability notes for the remainder of the year, he would be eligible to apply for full medical retirement. He also planned to apply for Social Security Disability and had decided that he would never return to work. Medical records revealed that he minimized his history of depression during the clinical interview and appeared to have developed major depressive disorder and a nonspecific anxiety disorder. While he attended a few sessions with a rehabilitation psychologist, these mostly focused on validation of his neurological symptoms as being due to concussion. His care was disproportionately provided in the medical realm despite no basis of a neurological cause for his myriad of persisting symptoms. His outpatient rehabilitation treatment included 27 physical therapy sessions, 27 occupational therapy sessions, and 16 speech therapy sessions. While there was no evidence of exaggerated emotional pathology on the exam via SVTs, his performances on various PVTs were profoundly low (e.g., below chance) and pervasive. There was evidence of significant overreporting of cognitive and somatic complaints on SVTs. He also presented with dramatically inconsistent grip strength over time and inconsistent visual field deficits that did not make sense clinically.

When Mr. X's physical therapist was initially asked if she had ever noticed any inconsistency in his presentation over time, she stated that he had always been very consistent. When it was pointed out to the physical therapist the next day that her own documentation showed inconsistent grip strength over time, she responded by saying that she was indeed aware of this but did not want to mention this to the examiner because she did not want it to look bad for the patient. She also responded that if a patient cries during a session when describing symptoms (as this patient did) the crying is considered evidence that the self-report is accurate and not to be questioned. She stated that she would bet her physical therapy license that Mr.

X would pass effort tests when he returned for the neuropsychological evaluation. These are troubling examples of an attempt by a rehabilitation team member to subvert an assessment by misrepresenting prior findings and an overreliance on subjective feelings to guide clinical decision-making and predictions of future outcomes.

When Mr. X returned for feedback, the "good news bad news" approach was employed. He and his significant other were also shown how he had performed much worse that a 9-year-old child on objectively simple tasks despite the fact that the child had severe brain tissue loss, chronic epilepsy, treatment with high-dose benzodiazepines, and mental retardation (Carone, 2014). It was also mentioned to him that his significant other told the examiner that she believed that he was capable of much more than he was doing prior to the assessment. It was explained to him that he appeared to be resigned to a disability role and that his examination results appeared to reflect purposeful suppression of performance. Weekly psychological counseling was suggested that actually addressed his underlying emotional problems and to help address his motivational problems so that he could become more functional. Mr. X expressed disagreement with the interpretation but did not have an alternative explanation for how his test performance could be so profoundly below expectations. He did not express any outward anger and left the office amicably once the session was concluded.

On the day of his next follow-up session with the rehabilitation nurse practitioner, it was reportedly explained to Mr. X that the test results showed that he "tanked" (i.e., did not try his best) on the examination. Regardless of the nurse practitioner agreeing with the validity testing results, no mention was made of this in the clinical note (it was later told to the neuropsychologist by the nurse practitioner); rather, the clinical note stated that Mr. X should continue to receive disability benefits based on his reported symptoms (even though the examination showed that his symptom reporting was invalid). On the same day, Mr. X delivered a complaint letter to the president of the hospital alleging that he was mistreated by the examiner (e.g., called "mentally retarded") and that the test results were incompetently interpreted. Hospital administration officials requested a response from the neuropsychologist, which included a blind interpretation by one of the PVT test publishers who turned out to be in agreement with the neuropsychologist's interpretation. A hospital patient satisfaction staff member reflexively sent a letter to Mr. X to apologize for the neuropsychologist's behavior. It was only after a subsequent meeting with higher-level hospital administration members (at the request of the neuropsychologist) to explain the nature and risks of evaluating malingering patients in a rehabilitation context that a clarifying letter was sent to the neuropsychologist stating that the original letter should not be interpreted as a verification of wrongdoing. A copy of the second letter was not sent to Mr. X because hospital administration officials stated that they did not want to anger him. Mr. X continued to receive disability notes from the rehabilitation treatment team.

The case of Mr. X highlights the complex challenges that can sometimes emerge when assessing patients who malinger in a rehabilitation setting and when providing feedback. Although feedback models exist to mitigate against hostile reactions, such reactions cannot be prevented in all cases and take many different shapes and forms, each of which have their own potential negative repercussions. Such cases also present a significant challenge to the rehabilitation team dynamic, especially if the exaggerated behavior is not detected until long after treatment has been initiated. Problems such as these can be reduced by incorporating validity assessment methods in the initial stage of patient contact in order to guide treatment. While there is an adage that many rehabilitation providers are treatment providers and not assessors, we do not believe that the two need to be mutually exclusive. Rather, a rehabilitation treatment plan should be guided and modified based on objective assessment results with an integration of validity results from within the same discipline or another discipline.

Case 3: Feedback in a Case of Genuine Neurological Impairment

Mrs. Z was a 53-year-old woman referred by her physiatrist for a neuropsychological evaluation which was performed 6 months after suffering two strokes: a small subacute lacunar stroke in the left cerebellar hemisphere and an infarct in the right parietal lobe. There was no pending litigation or compensation claim. A family member stated that she planned to hire a disability attorney in the future. She applied for Social Security Disability Insurance payments in the past and was rejected and was seeking a second opinion as to whether she was disabled. She returned to work 2 months after the strokes and reported difficulty completing her job duties. Her supervisor stated that she completed most of her job duties adequately but questioned her ability to respond to emergency situations because she seemed to get easily flustered in response to stress and had been known to *give up and walk away from challenging situations*. She acknowledged motivational problems and reported depression and anxiety. She had a high level of job dissatisfaction and chronic work stress. Results from cognitive testing showed a few mild to moderately low cognitive test scores (mostly in the area of executive functioning), good effort on some PVTs, and poor effort on a PVT that is designed to appear the most challenging.

While it was likely that some of Ms. Z's low test scores reflected damage from the stroke (e.g., verbal executive dysfunction due to damaged frontocerebellar connections), it was also concluded that her test performance did not reflect her full capabilities. While some of her low scores could have been impacted by a likely upcoming disability appeal, feedback focused on helping her understand how her tendency to disengage from situations she perceived to be stressful and challenging was causing problems for her. Her history of walking away from prior challenges at work was used as an analogy to help her explain what occurred at times during testing, and this comparison made those results easier for her to understand and accept. This information was also passed on to her rehabilitation treatment team so that a greater focus would be on helping her persist through challenges. It was concluded that she was not disabled from her job, which was mostly sedentary. She was referred for mental health counseling to help treat her depression, anxiety, and motivational problems.

Summary and Conclusions

There are many reasons for invalid data and presentations that are important for rehabilitation professionals to understand. While malingering is one possible explanation, it is not the only one, and healthcare providers also need to be mindful of underreporting. Management of invalid presentations involves establishing rapport, focusing on evidence-based data, remaining respectful during patient interactions, using the "good news bad news" approach, trying to identify precipitants, and referring for treatment as needed. There are differing perspectives on whether to use confrontational versus nonconfrontational approaches in managing invalid presentation, but we generally advocate for the use of *respectful* confrontation. More research is needed with larger samples to determine the efficacy of various management approaches for invalid presentations.

9 Forensic and Compensation-Seeking Applications of Validity Assessment in Rehabilitation Psychology and Settings

REHABILITATION PROFESSIONALS UNDERSTAND that some patients exaggerate symptoms to avoid attending therapies or returning to unpleasant or dangerous situations (e.g., work), to obtain drugs, or to receive unneeded services (e.g., factitious disorder). Whereas, other patients minimize symptoms to obtain passes for temporary leave from the hospital, seek discharge, maintain independence at home or with activities such as driving, or return to military service or other work due to a sense of duty or financial need. These motivations for patients who are providing misleading information or presentations can become a focus of clinical intervention. Rehabilitation professionals in general, and psychologists in particular, are commonly exposed to such cases during training, receive supervision, and through training and experience become prepared to address these challenging situations. In contrast, rehabilitation professionals may not be as prepared to address validity issues and other challenges that arise in the context of forensic matters.

Many patients undergo rehabilitation in the context of compensable injuries or illnesses and at some point pursue litigation and/or disability benefits. Personal injury litigation and administrative determinations of financial awards or benefits are typically considered forensic or medicolegal contexts (Bush, Demakis, & Rohling, 2017), despite psychological or other services being provided for clinical purposes. Whether a patient's injury or disability was caused by a motor vehicle collision, fall at work, military combat, or one of numerous other possible events that could result in compensation- or benefit-seeking actions by or on behalf of a patient, having the forensic context as the backdrop to the clinical services has important implications for the clinician. In some rehabilitation contexts, such as acute rehabilitation settings in which patients with severe impairments are evaluated and treated, clinicians typically have little knowledge of or interaction with forensic activities. However, in other rehabilitation settings, such as private practice or other outpatient settings, clinicians more routinely are asked by patients or their family members to complete paperwork or submit reports for disability benefits or are contacted directly by attorneys for information that will be used in personal injury litigation. Secondary gain contexts such as these offer incentive for patients to perform poorly on cognitive tests or to misrepresent their current symptoms or premorbid history. Family members often also have incentive to help maximize their loved one's financial award or benefits. In addition, in some clinical contexts, the clinician can have personal or financial incentive to assist patients and/or their representatives pursue their compensation or benefit goals. For example, the clinician may have a strong therapeutic connection with the patient and find it personally rewarding to offer assistance or advocate for the patient, thus having a bias in favor of the patient. Alternatively, the clinician who wants to increase forensic activities, and thus income, may have financial incentive to provide information or materials that will favor the patient's (and attorney's) case, thereby generating more forensic work. The link between forensic contexts and suboptimal performance or invalid responding is well established in the forensic psychology and neuropsychology literature. The primary goal of the present chapter is to help integrate that previously established information with rehabilitation practice.

Neurological Symptoms and Pain

Attorneys, triers of fact, and administrative financial decision makers typically seek information about a possible causal link between neurological signs and symptoms and an identified precipitating event, such as a motor vehicle collision. Rehabilitation records are often part of the information relied on for this purpose, and some rehabilitation professionals may be asked to offer opinions, in writing or via testimony, specifically on this issue. However, the ability to provide informed opinions that lead to just outcomes is often not as straightforward as it may seem. Even patients who have incontrovertible evidence of severe injuries sustained in a known accident can have premorbid (e.g., preinjury emotional and social functioning) or comorbid issues (intoxication at time of accident) that influence litigation and would need to be considered in order for just compensation to be provided. A rehabilitation professional who provides testimony about the causal link between a known accident, objectively established injuries, and persisting impairments without awareness or consideration of all relevant premorbid and comorbid factors does a disservice to the legal system and the parties involved in the legal matter, including the injured person.

Rehabilitation patients commonly report having headaches, dizziness, visual disturbances, memory problems, concentration problems, and other neurological problems. Such symptoms can serve as the foundation for the pursuit of financial compensation associated with established or suspected neurological injury. In such situations, patients have an incentive to overreport symptoms and attribute them to the compensable event. While these various neurological symptoms can result from neurological injury, they are also commonly experienced by persons with no history of brain trauma. That is, they are nonspecific. Lees-Haley and Brown (1993) found that 62% of outpatient family practice patients report having headaches and that 20% report having memory problems. Additionally, the physical symptoms (fatigue, dizzy spells), emotional symptoms (anger, impatience) and cognitive symptoms (memory and concentration problems) that constitute symptoms often attributed to "postconcussion syndrome" occur frequently in the normal population (Putnam & Millis, 1994). These symptoms increase in relation to stress, even for individuals without brain trauma (Gouvier et al., 1992). While uncertainty about the extent and timing of recovery following an injury can be stressful, litigation and the pursuit of benefits can add considerably to a patient's overall stress level, thereby increasing the scope or severity of symptoms.

Like neurological symptoms, significant pain can also result from injuries sustained in compensable events and can serve as the basis for litigation or pursuit of benefits. Also like neurological symptoms, pain is commonly experienced in the general population. More than 25 million adults in the United States experience daily, chronic pain, and more than 23 million experience considerable pain (Nahin, 2015). Despite the frequency of neurological symptoms and pain in the general population, there can be a tendency to attribute them to the event in question. Gunstad and Suhr (2001) noted, "Following any negative event, people may attribute all symptoms to that negative event (the "good old days" hypothesis)" (p. 323). This is the logical fallacy of *post hoc, ergo propter hoc.* Furthermore, the pursuit of compensation may influence the subjective expression of neurological symptoms following head injury (Feinstein et al., 2001).

Retrospective attribution of neurological symptoms to a possible neurological injury can also be misleading. Lees-Haley et al. (2001) found that 51% of their sample of litigating individuals with non-brain injuries reported feeling dazed immediately after the trauma, and 65% reported feeling confused. Thus, a temporal relationship between the onset of neurological symptoms and an accident does not necessarily imply the presence of a neurological injury. Therefore, clinicians making statements of causality regarding reported symptoms, whether in their records or statements to triers of fact or financial decision makers, should keep in mind the nonspecific nature of the symptoms, including the incentive to the patient to overreport symptoms, underreport preinjury problems, and misattribute symptoms to a compensable event.

Validity Assessment in Forensic Contexts

Invalid responding and performance are common in forensic contexts, with base rates ranging from a sizable minority (e.g., 30%) or to more than 50% in Veterans Administration contexts (review by Bush & Graver, 2013), Social Security Disability evaluation contexts (Chafetz, 2008), and civil litigation (Larrabee, 2007). Effort has been found to have a greater effect than severe brain injury on cognitive test performance for claimants seeking compensation (Green, Rohling, Lees-Haley, & Allen, 2001; Meyers, Volbrecht, Axelrod, & Reinsch-Boothby, 2011). Similarly, the prevalence of malingering in chronic pain patients with financial incentive is between 20% and 50%, with factors associated with the medicolegal context (e.g., the jurisdiction of a workers' compensation claim or attorney representation) associated with slightly higher malingering rates (Greve et al., 2009c). Likewise, symptom and performance validity assessment with litigants who have symptoms of posttraumatic stress disorder revealed that 29% failed at least one performance validity test (PVT) and that 48% failed at least one symptom validity test (SVT) (Demakis, Gervais, & Rohling, 2008). Mittenberg et al. (2002) reported a 30% base rate of malingering or symptom exaggeration for individuals with disability or workers' compensation cases. Thus, the likelihood that about one-third to one-half of patients in secondary gain contexts present in an invalid manner cannot be ignored.

In addition to overreporting symptoms, rehabilitation patients who are pursuing benefits or are involved in litigation may benefit from presenting their premorbid functioning as being better than it was before the compensable injury. Doing so helps to more clearly illustrate postinjury problems. Incorrect information of any type increases the challenges normally faced by clinicians who are striving to make accurate diagnoses and recommendations. For these reasons, relying solely on patient or family report can result in clinicians receiving incorrect and misleading information, which in turn can lead to incorrect diagnoses, statements of causality, prognostic determinations, and recommendations. Obtaining records of premorbid functioning and achievements (e.g., school transcripts, formal job descriptions, work evaluations, military records) allows clinicians to combine objective and self-reported information and to determine whether the information converges to provide a clear understanding of the patient's prior functioning or diverges and leaves uncertainty and doubts about response validity.

The ability of rehabilitation professionals to make statements that are of value to forensic decision makers—about cognitive and emotional functioning, including diagnosis, causality, prognosis, and ability to perform activities at home or in the community—requires that the patient respond honestly to background questions, put forth good effort on ability measures, and responded truthfully on measures of psychological functioning. However, opinions about validity cannot be based on clinical judgment alone (Guilmette, 2013). As explained earlier in this book (e.g., chapters 2 and 3), a multimethod approach to validity assessment should typically be used and appropriately interpreted. In litigation contexts in particular, there is a need to assess the veracity of both cognitive and psychological symptoms. The ability of administrators of compensation and benefit services to allocate resources in a just manner and the ability of triers of fact to reach just conclusions demands that the results provided by rehabilitation professionals be based on valid information and data.

Roles and Relationships

Differences exist in the roles rehabilitation professionals play and the nature of the services that are provided in clinical and forensic contexts. Because rehabilitation professionals are trained in clinical contexts, the differences between clinical and forensic practices are typically learned after completion of formal training, often unintentionally. Because some rehabilitation patients have compensable injuries or pursue disability benefits, clinical reports may be used by attorneys, administrative decision makers, or others to help support a legal position or inform forensic decisions. In such instances, rehabilitation professionals find themselves thrust into a forensic context and must learn what to expect, how professional behaviors may need to be altered, and what role needs to taken in a given case. Clarifying roles and expectations with patients, family members, referral sources, and attorneys is a very important aspect of ethical practice, as is practicing within the bounds of one's professional competence (American Psychological Association, 2010, 2013). Clinicians who do not feel adequately prepared to provide forensic reports or testimony, do not think doing so would be indicated in a given case, or simply have no interest in being involved in forensic matters should inform all involved parties at the outset. If a request for later forensic services can reasonably be anticipated at the outset of the rehabilitative services, the clinician should clarify what actions, if any, will be offered toward the pursuit of forensic goals. Conveying such information to prospective patients when first contacted, or including information of that nature in the informed consent process and documents, can help avoid confusion, frustration, and disappointment at a later date. In some cases, the patient may prefer to seek services elsewhere if it is made clear at the outset that the clinician does not want to testify or provide a forensic report in a legal matter.

Rehabilitation professionals, perhaps more than most healthcare specialists, advocate for their patients. Such advocacy helps patients obtain needed resources and materials, promotes functioning and well-being, and strengthens rapport between patients and clinicians. Rehabilitation professionals want to be helpful to their patients and their families and often develop strong positive feelings (while maintaining appropriate professional boundaries) for their patients. Experience suggests that, in general, rehabilitation professionals trust their patients and accept what their patients tell them and the manner in which they present at face value. Compared to some other specialties (e.g., pain management), there is relatively little professional skepticism on the part of rehabilitation professionals. This acceptance and desire to be helpful, while beneficial in some ways, can be detrimental to both patient care and forensic decisions if not handled in a measured way.

A clinician's well-intentioned desire to be helpful can be manipulated by patients such that patients' unverified statements of symptom severity and permanence, disability, and causality are translated into medical documents or testimony that are simply wrong and are misleading to forensic decision makers. For example, Wolfe (2000) reported that physicians who initially identified disability in an individual based on their clinical assessment subsequently admitted they had been misled after being shown evidence of the individual's intact function outside of the assessment. Wolfe stated, "physicians have a bias toward trust and empathy" (p. 1115), and so they are easily manipulated by clients. In addition, healthcare providers may be pressured on the telephone, in person, or via e-mail by a patient's attorney to support a particular position (e.g., that the motor vehicle collision is the cause of patient's symptoms) without evidence to support it. Rehabilitation professionals must be careful resist the temptation to accede to such improper requests based on a belief that advancing a patient's preferred legal outcome is synonymous with beneficent patient advocacy.

Much has been written in forensic psychology and neuropsychology about the importance of understanding the differences between clinical and forensic roles and striving to maintain clarity in one's professional roles (e.g., Bush & Morgan, 2017; Bush, Connell, & Denney, 2006). Maintaining role clarity and, typically, separation is needed because the goals and activities of clinical and forensic roles tend to conflict. For example, forensic decision makers seek information that is objective; however, rehabilitation professionals in their clinical roles typically have a bias in favor of their patients. They understandably want what is best for the patient with whom they have a strong helping relationship. However, attempting to conduct an objective examination or otherwise generate objective opinions when one has already established a position of treating clinician and patient advocate can threaten the scientific basis of one's conclusions, particularly in medicolegal contexts where litigation status influences manifestation of symptoms (Binder & Rohling, 1996; Feinstein et al., 2001).

Serving as both a treating clinician and a forensic expert for the same patient is an example of assuming conflicting roles that threaten to harm patient care and the pursuit of fair and appropriate litigation outcomes or benefit allocation. This separation of roles does not mean that clinicians do not and cannot have a role in forensic or administrative matters. Rather, it is the nature of the contribution to these processes that must be clarified, both within the clinician's mind and between the clinician and other involved parties, including the patient and attorney.

Clinicians can provide valuable information, in writing or testimony, about the facts of a patient's treatment and any evaluations on which such treatment is based. In such situations, clinicians should base their opinions and conclusions on the information they have obtained, limiting the confidence placed in their conclusions according to the amount and nature of the information that has been obtained.

In contrast to the treating clinician, the forensic expert typically gathers extensive records, beyond medical records; performs a comprehensive evaluation, including thorough validity assessment; and interviews collateral sources of information as needed. Based on such information, the forensic expert is well positioned to offer opinions and conclusions about proximate causes of the presenting problems, presence of and degree of impairment, and prognosis or permanency, often with a greater degree of accuracy and thus certainty than most treating doctors are in a position to offer. Treating doctors who may not have all relevant records or access to important collateral sources of information, or perform extensive testing, including validity assessment, do a disservice to forensic decision makers when they overstate their opinions and conclusions. Despite the desire to be helpful to the patient's cause, including concern that failure to be helpful in the forensic matter could adversely affect the treating relationship, treating clinicians must limit their opinions and testimony to clinical issues and avoid addressing the ultimate legal issue (*Specialty Guidelines for Forensic Psychology* [SGFP], Guideline 4.02.02, Expert Testimony by Practitioners Providing Therapeutic Services; APA, 2013). The SGFP define the provision of both treatment and forensic services to the same patient as a multiple relationship. Guideline 4.01.01 (Therapeutic-Forensic Role Conflicts) states: "Providing forensic and therapeutic psychological services to the same individual or closely related individuals involves multiple relationships that may impair objectivity and/or cause exploitation or other harm" (p. 11). The APA (2010) Ethics Code, Standard 3.06 (Conflicts of Interest) explains that when a clinician has a professional relationship (i.e., treating doctor) with a patient and then assumes a different professional role (i.e., forensic expert) with the same patient, the clinician's objectivity or effectiveness in performing the professional functions could be affected. A rehabilitation professional who has provided clinical services to a patient and is subsequently asked to provide a forensic report, a "narrative" report for forensic purposes, or testimony should clarify the limitations of such services or the reasons why the forensic services will not be provided.

Conclusions

Many rehabilitation patients pursue compensation and/or benefits for their injuries and persisting symptoms and limitations. Rehabilitation records are often part of the evidence supplied to decision makers to help in their determinations about whether compensation or benefits should be awarded to the patient. In addition, written opinions or testimony may be requested of the clinician to elaborate on or clarify information contained in the records. Clinicians can provide a valuable service by educating forensic decision makers about the clinical findings and treatment. However, clinicians commonly want to be helpful to the patient. The wish to be helpful to the patient in the forensic matter introduces bias into the forensic process, which can skew opinions and contribute to inappropriate and unfair legal decisions. Additionally, compared to forensic evaluations, most clinical evaluations are less comprehensive and do not assess validity as thoroughly. In forensic contexts in which invalid responding and performing are common, the combination of the clinician's bias toward the patient and the less comprehensive evaluation process limits the value of the clinician's opinions regarding forensic matters. In addition, treating clinicians who perform forensic services for their patients may threaten the treating relationship. For example, evaluation findings that are unhelpful to the patient's litigation or pursuit of benefits, such as suboptimal effort or ability testing that is within normal limits, can adversely affect the treating relationship. Rehabilitation professionals who are asked to provide information in forensic contexts should clarify with the patient and the requesting party (if other than the patient) the nature of the information that will be provided, based on an understanding of the relevant clinical and ethical issues, explaining the issues to the involved parties as needed.

10 Ethical Considerations Involving Validity Assessment in Rehabilitation Psychology and Settings

VALIDITY ASSESSMENT IN rehabilitation psychology and settings is based on the general bioethical principles of beneficence and nonmaleficence. For assessment results to be of value in the accurate understanding of the patient, and to avoid diagnoses, recommendations, or allocation of services or benefits that are unhelpful, harmful, or inappropriate, the results must be valid. Clinicians need to maintain an awareness that some patients, intentionally or unintentionally, overreport or underreport symptoms and functional limitations, underreport preinjury problems, and perform in a suboptimal manner on ability tests. As a result, validity assessment has become a standard of practice in neuropsychology contexts, and we believe that this should be the case in rehabilitation contexts as well. Because patient care and related decisions about patients rest on assessment results, clinicians have an ethical obligation to assess symptom and performance validity. The manner in which such assessment occurs varies based on the patient population and setting but typically consists of a multimethod approach that involves standardized validity assessment measures.

The goal of this chapter is to describe ethical and professional issues underlying validity assessment in rehabilitation psychology and settings. Case examples are used, and principles and standards from the 2010 APA Ethics Code are emphasized.

Case 1: The Bouncing Phone

A 30-year-old man sustained injuries to his back, including herniated discs in the cervical and lumbar spine, when he fell from a ladder at work 6 months ago. He is seen by a rehabilitation psychologist because of severe adjustment-related depression and anxiety resulting from the accident, injuries, pain, and functional limitations. During the initial appointment, the man, who ambulates with a cane and wears a cervical collar, tells the psychologist that he had no emotional problems before the accident but now is very distressed because he cannot perform basic activities such as tying his shoes, picking up after his dog, or doing the dishes because he cannot bend or look down. He is tearful as he describes the changes in his life. After the interview portion of the appointment, the psychologist administers the Minnesota Multiphasic Personality Inventory-2nd Edition-Restructured Form (MMPI-2-RF) on the computer, and the report is immediately available. The results of the validity scales are within normal limits, and the clinical scale elevations are consistent with the reported depression and anxiety. The patient and psychologist establish a plan for psychotherapy. The patient leaves the office. The psychologist has a few minutes before the next appointment and takes the opportunity to look out the window at the beautiful spring day. As the psychologist looks across the parking lot, the patient is seen walking nimbly without using his cane. As he starts to climb into his pickup truck, he drops his phone and quickly bends to scoop it up as it bounces on the pavement. He does not appear to be in any type of pain or discomfort. He then climbs into the truck without incident and drives away. The psychologist is a bit puzzled by the patient's agility but does not give it much thought in the context of the valid MMPI-2-RF profile. The psychologist discounts the behavioral observations and looks forward to treating the man's emotional adjustment problems.

Psychologists have an ethical obligation to base their work on the scientific and professional knowledge of the discipline (Ethical Standard 2.04, Bases for Scientific and Professional Judgments). As has been emphasized throughout this book, optimal validity assessment is a multimethod process. The assessment techniques used must be sufficient to substantiate the findings, recommendations, and plans (Ethical Standard 9.01, Bases for Assessments). While standardized, psychometric symptom validity assessment is typically an essential part of that process, behavioral observations are also an integral component. In this case, the psychologist selected and used an appropriate psychological test but completely discounted compelling evidence of symptom overreporting obtained through observation of the patient's behavior outside of the office setting. Despite finding the patient's behavior a bit puzzling, the psychologist gave all weight to the MMPI-2-RF results, thus missing the opportunity to reconsider the treatment plan or at least gather more information.

There are instances in which conflicting evidence from different sources may need to be weighed, with final determinations being more consistent with one piece of evidence than another, but in this case an essential piece of evidence was summarily discounted. Even though the observations occurred outside of the psychologist's office, they were still visible from the psychologist's office setting and are within the proper ethical bounds to document. By ignoring the relevant behavioral observations, the resulting treatment plan is likely to waste valuable resources, be unhelpful to the patient, and lead to unjust administrative decisions. Because the validity assessment process can be ongoing in situations in which the patient and clinician continue to interact, a vigilant psychologist during the course of treatment will have the opportunity to continue to monitor the patient's veracity and alter conclusions and plans as additional information becomes available.

Case 2: This Cannot Be Explained Away

A 45-year-old woman who sustained third-degree burns on her lower extremities in a motor vehicle collision is receiving inpatient rehabilitation. She is referred to a psychologist for treatment of depression as well as reports of memory and concentration problems. During the initial consultation, the patient reported having significant problems with focus and remembering information, but her cognition appeared grossly intact to the psychologist. Based on this discrepancy between reported and observed cognition, the psychologist decides to perform a brief cognitive evaluation and includes the Test of Memory Malingering (TOMM) (Tombaugh, 1996). The patient performs very poorly across cognitive domains and achieves a TOMM Trial 2 score of 17 out of 50. Conceptualizing the case from a biopsychosocial perspective, the psychologist concludes that the patient has severe cognitive problems that result from a combination of the patient's pain, pain medications, poor sleep, depression, and the effects of a possible concussion sustained in the collision. That combination of issues is also believed to result in the very low TOMM score. The psychologist understands that there could be a lawsuit as a result of the collision but does not want to contaminate the therapeutic alliance by asking the patient or her family about litigation at this point. The psychologist recommends continued treatment of the various factors that seem to be impacting the patient's cognition as well as strategies and techniques to help compensate for the cognitive problems.

Psychologists have an ethical responsibility to interpret test results in a manner consistent with the empirical evidence supporting use of the test with various populations (i.e., test factors), as well as situational and personal characteristics of the patient (Ethical Standard 9.06, Interpreting Assessment Results). As with tests of psychological functioning and cognitive abilities, the results of validity assessment measures should be compared to appropriate normative groups, but they can also be interpreted according to the statistical probability of obtaining a given score. More specifically, performance validity test (PVT) results should be compared to known patient and/or research groups, and forced-choice PVTs (e.g., the TOMM) should be interpreted in a manner consistent with the binomial theorem. In this case, the psychologist failed to accurately interpret the TOMM results. A score of 17 is not only below generally accepted cutoff scores and is not only below chance, it is *significantly below* chance. Statistically speaking, the only plausible way for the patient to achieve a score of 17 is to know the correct answer and to intentionally choose the incorrect option. While this patient is experiencing multiple issues that could affect cognitive performance, those issues could not result in a TOMM Trial 2 score of 17. Because the patient achieved a score on the TOMM that is significantly below chance, the results of the cognitive ability tests cannot be accepted as valid. Thus, the psychologist's failure to understand this basic interpretation fact is likely to result in a misunderstanding of the patient's abilities and clinical needs and misdirected clinical resources.

Case 3: No Boat Rocking

A psychologist begins working in an outpatient rehabilitation program performing cognitive evaluations of patients who have sustained injuries in athletic events or accidents in any context. The rehabilitation program generates good income for the hospital by performing brief cognitive evaluations, engaging patients in biweekly computer-based cognitive rehabilitation programs, and referring patients for other extensive rehabilitation therapy services and additional diagnostic tests. As a result, the program manager is held in high regard by the higher administration. The new psychologist observes that no validity assessment measures are used as part of the test battery or by any of the other rehabilitation staff, and the program does not seem to consider potential differences between patients injured in noncompensable contexts (e.g., amateur athletes) and those who may benefit financially or through avoidance of unwanted responsibilities from their injuries. In fact, inquiring about litigation and other compensation status is a matter that none of the rehabilitation therapists have been trained to ask about or consider. The psychologist is excited to be able to offer some suggestions to the program manager to help improve the services that the program provides. In a meeting with the manager she outlines ways to integrate into the assessment process validity assessment measures and procedures that will add little time to the assessment and will generate very valuable data for guiding treatment, as well as identifying those who are not appropriate for the program. She also recommends two separate patient tracks, one for patients who were not injured in compensable contexts and one for those who were. She provides position statements, research articles, and other evidence to support the value of her suggestions. The program manager is unwilling to consider either proposal with the explanation that use of failed validity assessment results will be difficult to explain to patients in a clinical context, will be difficult to reconcile with the staff's view about the veracity of patient self-report, and runs the risk of patients becoming upset due to feeling that that they are being accused of lying. These factors could make it more difficult to justify the need for ongoing assessments and therapy and can lead some patients to drop out of the program, which could have significant financial implications. The manager indicates that the program is successful as is and that there is no need to rock the boat by implementing any changes, and suggests that the psychologist not use validity assessment techniques at all. The manager is not open to any additional discussion.

Psychologists delivering services as employees of, or consultants to, organizations may confront challenges to practicing in a manner that they consider most appropriate. Threats to optimal or preferred rehabilitation practices from within the organization can occur for many reasons, such as (1) the organization has limited resources (e.g., financial, space, personnel), (2) scope of practice overlap among professions (i.e., turf issues) is inadequately addressed, (3) supervisors or administrators do not fully appreciate best practices in psychology and therefore choose not to allocate more resources or make programmatic changes; or (4) supervisors or administrators are aware that preferred practices are attainable but elect not to make improvements because the status quo is advantageous to them and/or the organization.

In some instances, organization practices may conflict with ethical responsibilities. A policy on psychological assessment that denies the clinician the ability to select, use, and interpret tests in a manner that reflects best practices is inconsistent with ethical practice (Ethical Standards 9.01, Bases of Assessments; 9.02, Use of Assessments; 9.06,

Interpreting Assessment Results) and puts the clinician in an ethical bind. Consistent with ethical practice (General Principle A, Beneficence and Nonmaleficence; Ethical Standard 3.04 Avoiding Harm), the results of evaluations are most likely to be helpful and least likely to be harmful to patients when an appropriate test battery is used and the results are interpreted in an evidence-based manner. Denying clinicians the ability to perform appropriate evaluations as described by national professional organizations and interpret the results in an evidence-based manner poses a conflict for clinicians. According to Ethical Standard 1.03 (Conflicts between Ethics and Organizational Demands), when psychologists experience a conflict between the requirements of the work setting and those of professional ethics, they should clarify the nature of the conflict, make known their commitment to professional ethics, and take reasonable steps to resolve the conflict. Standard 10.10 (Test Interpretation) of the Standards for Educational and Psychological Testing (American Educational Research Association, American Psychological Association, and National Council on Measurement in Education, 2014) states that those who select tests and interpret test results should not allow others (including employers) who have a vested interest in the outcome of the assessment to have an inappropriate influence on the interpretation of the assessment results. Although this standard focuses on not allowing employers or others to influence test interpretation, it is equally important that those with a vested interest in the outcome of the assessment do not inappropriately influence test selection or use when such influence is inconsistent with best practices.

The psychologist in this case followed the recommended course of action for someone experiencing a conflict between organization and ethical requirements, to no avail. In such cases, it is important for psychologists to seek the advice and counsel of colleagues and to document the results of those discussions. Such discussions typically result in generating useful options for dealing with the situation. It would be unethical for the psychologist to practice as instructed. The psychologist should either leave the position or continue to practice in an ethical manner. If the latter is chosen, the psychologist can hope for a change in leadership while persisting with efforts to make positive changes within the organization and within the profession, try to reopen a discussion with the manager in the future, and use a combination of collegial support, relevant professional position papers, and consensus conference statements if asked to defend her current practice decisions to higher administration officials.

Case 4: Suboptimal Competence

A rehabilitation psychologist employed by the Veterans Administration (VA) consults with a subacute rehabilitation program that is housed in a VA community living center (i.e., a long-term care facility). He understands the importance of validity assessment and emphasizes its importance to trainees. He learns from a listserv posting that there is a performance validity index that can be calculated from the brief neuropsychological test that he commonly uses with the subacute rehabilitation patients (Repeatable Battery for the Assessment of Neuropsychological Status [RBANS]; Randolph, 1998). He finds that the RBANS Effort Index (EI; Silverberg, Wertheimer, and Fichtenberg, 2007) is easily calculated from the raw scores of two of the subtests, with cutoff scores obtained from the authors' original article. He and his trainees begin using the EI, and he is surprised to find that more than half of the patients are obtaining scores in the range considered "suspicious" for suboptimal performance. Nevertheless, knowing that clinical judgment alone tends to be insufficient for determinations of performance validity and that psychometric findings are often more informative, he considers all of the RBANS data invalid for those cases with EI scores in the invalid range. The trainees follow their mentor's practices. Within a few months, the psychologist experiences a substantial decline in the number of referrals for neuropsychological evaluations and is not sure why.

Performance validity research continues to evolve at a remarkable pace, and staying abreast of updated research for all of the specific tests employed in a rehabilitation psychology practice can be a time-consuming endeavor. Often, initial findings and cutoff scores for one patient population are not readily transferable to another population. After a performance validity test's initial publication or an embedded indicator's initial validation studies, considerable time may lapse before the results of replication or additional studies are published. Some such studies may not come to the attention of busy clinicians who use the measure. Thus, even well-intentioned and otherwise competent clinicians can make significant mistakes in some instances, with harmful effects for the patient's rehabilitation.

The psychologist in this case was unaware of subsequent research demonstrating (1) the weaknesses of the EI with cognitively impaired, medically ill, older adults (Hook et al., 2009); (2) the existence of the Effort Scale (Novitski et al., 2012), developed to overcome some of the weaknesses evident with the EI; and (3) a study comparing the EI and ES which found that "the ES may have more clinical utility when an individual has moderate or severe cognitive impairment and the EI may have more clinical utility when an individual has mild impairment in cognitive functioning" (Dunham et al., 2014; p. 639). This lack of awareness reflects suboptimal ethical practice. The psychologist's actions were inconsistent with competent practice in general (Ethical Standard 2.03, Maintaining Competence) and, more specifically, with Ethical Standards 9.01 (Bases for Assessments), 9.02 (Use of Assessments), and 9.06 (Interpreting Assessment Results). Although it is unrealistic for clinicians to be familiar with every article published on every test that they use, it is reasonable for clinicians to be familiar with relevant articles about a validity assessment measure when only a couple have been published and available for at least a couple of years.

Additionally, by not fully educating the trainees about validity assessment using the RBANS, the psychologist failed to facilitate competent practice by his trainees and thus failed to supervise in a competent manner (Ethical Standard 2.05, Delegation of Work to Others). The psychologist's practices seemed to adversely affect the reputation of psychology with the interdisciplinary team, resulting in reduced referrals for psychological evaluations for a patient population that was likely in need. This psychologist may have readily updated his practices if these issues were brought to his attention, but oftentimes such practices go unnoticed or unreported, to the detriment of all involved. Clinicians are well served by striving to remain abreast of the published literature on the assessment measures that they use. Setting up specific "alerts" from relevant journals can be part of the approach used to maintain awareness of publications of interest and, more generally, to maintain professional competence. Regular monitoring of professional listserv postings is another excellent way to keep up to date with relevant research.

Conclusions

Validity assessment is a standard of practice, and a multimethod, evidence-based approach to validity assessment is consistent with ethical practice. Rehabilitation settings and populations vary regarding the nature and extent of psychological assessment that is indicated in general, as well as the nature and extent of validity assessment. Given that even low-functioning patients and those near both ends of the developmental spectrum tend to perform well on PVTs, and that known group comparisons are available for many PVTs and patient populations, use of psychometric methods can and typically should be part of the validity assessment process for most rehabilitation patients. Obtaining evidence for or against a valid approach to psychological evaluations helps position clinicians to make accurate diagnoses and helpful recommendations and to inform decision makers about the best use of resources.

Consistent with positive ethics (Knapp, VandeCreek, & Fingerhut, 2017) and the 4 A's of ethical practice (Bush, 2009), *aspiring* to high standards of ethical practice involves *anticipating* challenges to appropriate validity assessment, *avoiding* pitfalls that can interfere with successful implementation of validity assessment, and *addressing* challenges and hurdles when they are encountered. Open exchanges—receiving as well as giving—of information within and across disciplines provides the greatest potential for informed clinicians to understand and meet the needs of patients, those assisting and caring for patients, and society.

References

Al-Ashkar, F., Mehra, R., & Mazzone, P. J. (2003). Interpreting pulmonary function tests: Recognize the pattern, and the diagnosis will follow. *Cleveland Clinic Journal of Medicine, 70,* 866, 868, 871–863, passim.
American Academy of Clinical Neuropsychology (AACN). (2007). American Academy of Clinical Neuropsychology (AACN) practice guidelines for neuropsychological assessment and consultation. *Clinical Neuropsychologist, 21,* 209–231.
American Educational Research Association, American Psychological Association, & National Council on Measurement in Education. (2014). *Standards for educational and psychological testing.* Washington, DC: American Educational Research Foundation.
American Psychiatric Association. (2013). *Diagnostic and statistical manual of mental disorders, 5th edition: DSM-5.* Arlington, VA: American Psychiatric Publishing.
American Psychological Association. (2010). *Ethical principles of psychologists and code of conduct.* http://www.apa.org/ethics/code/index.aspx
American Psychological Association. (2013). Specialty guidelines for forensic psychology. *American Psychologist, 68,* 7–19.
Amlani, A., Grewal, G. S., & Feldman, M. D. (2016). Malingering by proxy: A literature review and current perspectives. *Journal of Forensic Sciences, 61*(Suppl 1), S171–S176.
An, K. Y., Zakzanis, K. K., & Joordens, S. (2012). Conducting research with non-clinical healthy undergraduates: Does effort play a role in neuropsychological test performance? *Archives of Clinical Neuropsychology, 27,* 849–857.
Anastasi, A., & Urbina, S. (1997). *Psychological testing* (2nd ed.). New Jersey: Prentice Hall.
Archer, R. P., Handel, R. W., Ben-Porath, Y. S., & Tellegen, A. (2016). *Minnesota Multiphasic Personality Inventory-Adolescent-Restructured Form (MMPI-A RF): Administration, scoring, interpretation, and technical manual.* Minneapolis: University of Minnesota Press.

Armistead-Jehle, P., & Denney, R. L. (2015). The detection of feigned impairment using the WMT, MSVT, and NV-MSVT. *Applied Neuropsychology: Adult, 22*, 147–155.

Armistead-Jehle, P., Gervais, R. O., & Green, P. (2012a). Memory Complaints Inventory and symptom validity test performance in a clinical sample. *Archives of Clinical Neuropsychology, 27*, 725–734.

Armistead-Jehle, P., Gervais, R. O., & Green, P. (2012b). Memory Complaints Inventory results as a function of symptom validity test performance. *Archives of Clinical Neuropsychology, 27*, 101–113.

Armistead-Jehle, P., Grills, C. E., Bieu, R. K., & Kulas, J. F. (2016). Clinical utility of the memory complaints inventory to detect invalid test performance. *Clinical Neuropsychologist, 30*, 610–628.

Armistead-Jehle, P., Lange, B. J., & Green, P. (2016). Comparison of neuropsychological and balance performance validity testing. *Applied Neuropsychology: Adult*, 1–8.

Arnett, P. A. (2013). Introduction to secondary influences on neuropsychological test performance. In P. A. Arnett (Ed.), *Secondary influences on neuropsychological test performance* (pp. 1–3). New York, NY: Oxford University Press.

Ashendorf, L., Constantinou, M., & McCaffrey, R. J. (2004). The effect of depression and anxiety on the TOMM in community-dwelling older adults. *Archives of Clinical Neuropsychology, 19*, 145–159.

Baik, J. S., & Lang, A. E. (2007). Gait abnormalities in psychogenic movement disorders. *Movement Disorders, 22*, 395–399.

Bannwarth, B. (1999). Risk-benefit assessment of opioids in chronic noncancer pain. *Drug Safety, 21*, 283–296.

Barhon, L. I., Batchelor, J., Meares, S., Chekaluk, E., Shores, E. A. (2015). A comparison of the degree of effort involved in the TOMM and the ACS Word Choice Test using a dual-task paradigm. *Applied Neuropsychology: Adult, 22*, 114–123.

Barker, M. D., Horner, M. D., & Bachman, D. L. (2010). Embedded indices of effort in the repeatable battery for the assessment of neuropsychological status (RBANS) in a geriatric sample. *The Clinical Neuropsychologist, 24*, 1964–1077.

Bass, C., & Glaser, D. (2014). Early recognition and management of fabricated or induced illness in children. *Lancet, 383*, 1412–1421.

Bass, C., & Halligan, P. (2014). Factitious disorders and malingering: Challenges for clinical assessment and management. *Lancet, 383*, 1422–1432.

Bass, C., & Halligan, P. (2017). Factitious disorders and malingering in relation to functional neurologic disorders. *Handbook of Clinical Neurology, 139*, 509–520.

Bauer, L., O'Bryant, S. E., Lynch, J. K., McCaffrey, R. J., & Fisher, J. M. (2007). Examining the Test of Memory Malingering Trial 1 and Word Memory Test Immediate Recognition as screening tools for insufficient effort. *Assessment, 14*, 215–222.

Bayard, S., Adnet Bonte, C., Nibbio, A., & Moroni, C. (2007). [Memory symptom exaggeration in a patient with progressive multiple sclerosis outside any medico-legal context]. *Revue Neurologique, 163*, 730–733.

Behrouz, R., & Benbadis, S. R. (2014). Psychogenic pseudostroke. *Journal of Stroke and Cerebrovascular Diseases, 23*, e243–e248.

Benedict, R. H. (1997). *Brief Visuospatial Memory Test–Revised: Professional manual*. Odessa, FL: Psychological Assessment Resources.

Benedict, R. H., & Zivadinov, R. (2011). Risk factors for and management of cognitive dysfunction in multiple sclerosis. *Nature Reviews: Neurology, 7,* 332–342.

Ben-Porath, Y. S. (2012). *Interpreting the MMPI-2-RF.* Minneapolis: University of Minnesota Press.

Ben-Porath, Y. S. (2013). *Using the MMPI-2-RF validity scales in forensic assessments.* Retrieved March 23, 2017, from http://www.apadivisions.org/division-18/publications/newsletters/gavel/2013/07/forensic-assessments.aspx

Ben-Porath, Y. S., & Tellegen, A. (2008). *MMPI-2-RF (Minnesota Multiphasic Personality Inventory-2 Restructured Form): Manual for administration, scoring, and interpretation.* Minneapolis: University of Minnesota Press.

Bianchini, K. J., Etherton, J. L., Greve, K. W., Henley, M. T., & Meyers, J. E. (2008). Classification accuracy of MMPI-2 validity scales in the detection of pain-related malingering: A known groups study. *Assessment, 15,* 435–449.

Bianchini, K. J., Greve, K. W., & Glynn, G. (2005). On the diagnosis of malingered pain-related disability: Lessons from cognitive malingering research. *Spine Journal, 5,* 404–417.

Bianchini, K. J., Mathias, C. W., & Greve, K. W. (2001). Symptom validity testing: A critical review. *Clinical Neuropsychologist, 15,* 19–45.

Binder, L. M. (1992). Malingering detected by forced choice testing of memory and tactile sensation: A case report. *Archives of Clinical Neuropsychology, 7,* 155–163.

Binder, L. M. (1993). Assessment of malingering after mild head trauma with the Portland Digit Recognition Test. *Journal of Clinical and Experimental Neuropsychology, 15,* 170–182.

Binder, L. M., & Campbell, K. A. (2004). Medically unexplained symptoms and neuropsychological assessment. *Journal of Clinical and Experimental Neuropsychology, 26,* 369–392.

Binder, L. M., & Rohling, M. L. (1996). Money matters: A meta-analytic review of the effects of financial incentives on recovery after closed head injury. *American Journal of Psychiatry, 153,* 5–8.

Binder, L. M., Storzbach, D., Campbell, K. A., Rohlman, D. S., Anger, W. K., & Members of the Portland Environmental Hazards Research Center. (2001). Neurobehavioral deficits associated with chronic fatigue syndrome in veterans with Gulf War unexplained illnesses. *Journal of the International Neuropsychological Society, 7,* 835–839.

Blaskewitz, N., Merten, T., & Kathmann, N. (2008). Performance of children on symptom validity tests: TOMM, MSVT, and FIT. *Archives of Clinical Neuropsychology, 23,* 379–391.

Bowden, S. C. (2017). Why do we need evidence-based neuropsychological practice? In S. C. Bowden (Ed.), *Neuropsychological assessment in the age of evidence-based practice: Diagnostic and treatment evaluations* (pp. 1–14). New York, NY: Oxford University Press.

Boone, K. B., Lu, P., Sherman, D., Palmer, B., Back, C., Shamieh, E., Warner-Chacon, K., & Berman, N. G. (2000). Validation of a new technique to detect malingering of cognitive symptoms: the b Test. *Archives of Clinical Neuropsychology, 15,* 227–241.

Boone, K. B. (2007). *Assessment of feigned cognitive impairment: A neuropsychological perspective.* New York: Guilford Press.

Boone, K. B. (2009). The need for continuous and comprehensive sampling of effort/response bias during neuropsychological examinations. *Clinical Neuropsychologist, 23,* 729–741.

Boone, K. B. (2013). *Clinical practice of forensic neuropsychology: An evidence-based approach.* New York, NY: Guilford Press.

Boone, K. B., Lu, P., Back, C., King, C., Lee, A., Philpott, L., ... Warner-Chacon, K. (2002). Sensitivity and specificity of the Rey Dot Counting Test in patients with suspect effort and various clinical samples. *Archives of Clinical Neuropsychology, 17,* 625–642.

Boone, K. B., Lu, P., & Herzberg, D. S. (2002a). *The b Test manual*. Los Angeles, CA: Western Psychological Services.

Boone, K. B., Lu, P., & Herzberg, D. S. (2002b). *The Dot Counting Test manual*. Los Angeles, CA: Western Psychological Services.

Boone, K. B., Salazar, X., Lu, P., Warner-Chacon, K., & Razani, J. (2002). The Rey 15-item recognition trial: A technique to enhance sensitivity of the Rey 15-item memorization test. *Journal of Clinical and Experimental Neuropsychology, 24*, 561–573.

Brandt, J., & Benedict, R. H. (2001). *Hopkins Verbal Learning Test—Revised: Professional Manual*. Lutz, FL.: Psychological Assessment Resources.

Brenner, L. A., Betthauser, L. M., Bahraini, N., Lusk, J. L., Terrio, H., Scher, A. I., & Schwab, K. A. (2015). Soldiers retruning from deployment: A qualitative study regarding exposure, coping and reintegration. *Rehabilitation Psychology, 60*, 277–285.

Brey, R. L., Hilliday, S. L., Saklad, A. R., Navarrete, M. G., Hermosillo-Romo, D., Stallworth, C. L., . . . McGlasson, D. (2002). Neuropsychiatric syndromes in lupus. *Neurology, 58*, 1214–1220.

British Psychological Society. (2009). *Assessment of effort in clinical testing of cognitive functioning for adults*. Leicester, UK: British Psychological Society.

Brooks, B. L. (2012). Victoria Symptom Validity Test performance in children and adolescents with neurological disorders. *Archives of Clinical Neuropsychology, 27*, 858–868.

Brooks, B. L., Ploetz, D. M., & Kirkwood, M. W. (2016). A survey of neuropsychologists' use of validity tests with children and adolescents. *Child Neuropsychology, 22*, 1001–1020.

Bruns, D., & Disorbio, J. M. (2003). *Battery for Health Improvement-2 manual*. Minneapolis, MN: Pearson.

Bruns, D., & Disorbio, J. M. (2014). The psychological evaluation of patients with chronic pain: a review of BHI 2 clinical and forensic interpretive considerations. *Psychological Injury and Law, 7*, 335–361.

Burton, R. L., Enright, J., O'Connell, M. E., Lanting, S., & Morgan, D. (2015). RBANS embedded measures of suboptimal effort in dementia: effort scale has a lower failure rate than the effort index. *Archives of Clinical Neuropsychology, 30*, 1–6.

Buscichio, K., Tiersky, L. A., DeLuca, J., & Natelson, B. H. (2004). Neuropsychological deficits in patients with chronic fatigue syndrome. *Journal of the International Neuropsychological Society, 10*, 278–285.

Bush, S. S. (2009). *Geriatric mental health ethics: A casebook*. New York, NY: Springer.

Bush, S. S. (2014). Assessing symptom and performance validity in veterans. In S. S. Bush (Ed.), *Psychological assessment of veterans* (pp. 433–452). New York, NY: Oxford University Press.

Bush, S. S., Allen, R. A., & Molinari, V. A. (2017). *Ethical practice in geropsychology*. Washington, DC: American Psychological Association.

Bush, S. S., & Bass, C. (2015). Assessment of validity with polytrauma veteran populations. *NeuroRehabilitation, 36*, 451–462.

Bush, S. S., Connell, M. A., & Denney, R. L. (2006). *Ethical practice in forensic psychology: A systematic model for decision making*. Washington, DC: American Psychological Association.

Bush, S. S., Demakis, G. J., & Rohling, M. L. (Eds.). (2017). Introduction. *APA handbook of forensic neuropsychology* (pp. xvii–xxii). Washington, DC: American Psychological Association Press.

Bush, S. S., & Graver, C. (2013). Symptom validity assessment of military and veteran populations following mild traumatic brain injury. In D. A. Carone & S. S. Bush (Eds.), *Mild traumatic brain injury: Symptom validity assessment and malingering* (pp. 381–397). New York: Springer Publishing Company.

Bush, S. S., Heilbronner, R. L., & Ruff, R. M. (2014). Psychological assessment of symptom and performance validity, response bias, and malingering: Official position of the Association for Psychological Advancement in Psychological Injury and Law. *Psychological Injury and Law, 7*, 197–205.

Bush, S. S., & Morgan, J. E. (2012). Improbable neuropsychological presentations: Assessment, diagnosis, and management. In S. S. Bush (Ed.), *Neuropsychological practice with veterans* (pp. 27–43). New York: Springer Publishing Company.

Bush, S. S., & Morgan, J. (2017). Ethical practice in forensic neuropsychology. In S. S. Bush, G. J. Demakis, & M. L. Rohling (Eds.), *APA handbook of forensic neuropsychology* (pp. 23–37). Washington, DC: American Psychological Association Press.

Bush, S. S., Ruff, R., Troster, A., Barth, J., Koffler, S., Pliskin, N., . . . Silver, C. (2005). Symptom validity assessment: Practice issues and medical necessity NAN policy and planning committee. *Archives of Clinical Neuropsychology, 20*, 419–426.

Bush, S. S., & Rush, B. K. (in press). Assessment. In R. G. Frank, T. R. Elliott, B. Caplan, L. Brenner, & S. Reid-Arndt (Eds.), *Handbook of rehabilitation psychology* (3rd ed.). Washington, DC: American Psychological Association.

Butcher, J. N., Dahlstrom, W. G., Graham, J. R., Tellegen, A., & Kaemmer, B. (1989). *Manual for administration and scoring the Minnesota Multiphasic Personality Inventory-2*. Minneapolis: University of Minnesota Press.

Butcher, J. N., Williams, C. L., Graham, J. R., Archer, R. P., Tellegen, A., Ben-Porath, Y. S., & Kaemmer, B. (1992). *MMPI-A: Manual for administration, scoring, and interpretation*. Minneapolis: University of Minnesota Press.

Camara, W. J., Nathan, J. S., & Puente, A. E. (2000). Psychological test usage: Implications in professional psychology. *Professional Psychology: Research and Practice, 31*, 141–154.

Carone, D. A. (2008). Children with moderate/severe brain damage/dysfunction outperform adults with mild-to-no brain damage on the Medical Symptom Validity Test. *Brain Injury, 22*, 960–971.

Carone, D. A. (2009). Test review of the Medical Symptom Validity Test. *Applied Neuropsychology, 16*.

Carone, D. A. (2013). Strategies for non-neuropsychology clinicians to detect noncredible presentations after mild traumatic brain injury. In D. A. Carone & S. S. Bush (Eds.), *Mild traumatic brain injury: Symptom validity assessment and malingering* (pp. 183–202). New York, NY: Springer.

Carone, D. A. (2014). Young child with severe brain volume loss easily passes the word memory test and medical symptom validity test: Implications for mild TBI. *Clinical Neuropsychologist, 28*, 146–162.

Carone, D. (2018). Understanding the role of medical and psychological iatrogenesis in neuropsychological assessment. In: J. E. Morgan & J. Ricker (Eds.), *Textbook of Clinical Neuropsychology* (2nd ed.). New York, NY: Routledge.

Carone, D. A. (2015). Chronic disability determination after work-related mild traumatic brain injury: Ethical problems and resolutions. *Journal of Head Trauma Rehabilitation, 30*, 228–230.

Carone, D. A. (2015a). Assessment of response bias in neurocognitive evaluations. *NeuroRehabilitation, 36*, 387–400.

Carone, D. A. (2015b). Clinical strategies to assess the credibility of presentations in children. In M. W. Kirkwood (Ed.), *Validity testing in child and adolescent assessment: Evaluating exaggeration, feigning, and non-credible effort* (pp. 107–124). New York, NY: Guilford Press.

Carone, D. A., & Bush, S. B. (Eds.). (2013). *Mild traumatic brain injury: Symptom validity assessment and malingering.* New York, NY: Springer.

Carone, D. A., Bush, S. S., & Iverson, G. L. (2013). Providing feedback on symptom validity, mental health, and treatment in mild traumatic brain injury. In D. A. Carone & S. S. Bush (Eds.), *Mild traumatic brain injury: Symptom validity assessment and malingering.* New York, NY: Springer.

Carone, D. A., Green, P., & Drane, D. L. (2014). Word Memory Test profiles in two cases with surgical removal of the left anterior hippocampus and parahippocampal gyrus. *Applied Neuropsychology: Adult, 21,* 155–160.

Carone, D. A., Iverson, G. L., & Bush, S. S. (2010). A model to approaching and providing feedback to patients regarding invalid test performance in clinical neuropsychological evaluations. *Clinical Neuropsychologist, 24,* 759–778.

Cashel, M. L., Rogers, R., Sewell, K., & Martin-Cannici, C. (1995). The Personality Assessment Inventory and the detection of defensiveness. *Assessment, 2,* 333–342.

Cassar, J. R., Hales, E. S., Longhurst, J. G., & Weiss, G. S. (1996). Can disability benefits make children sicker? *Journal of the American Academy of Child and Adolescent Psychiatry, 35,* 700–701.

Chafetz, M. D. (2008). Malingering on the Social Security disability consultative examination: Predictors and base rates. *Clinical Neuropsychologist, 22,* 529–546.

Chafetz, M. D., Abrahams, J. P., & Kohlmaier, J. (2007). Malingering on the Social Security disability consultative exam: a new rating scale. *Archives of Clinical Neuropsychology, 22,* 1–14.

Chafetz, M. D., & Biondolillo, A. (2012). Validity issues in Atkins death cases. *Clinical Neuropsychologist, 26,* 1358–1376.

Chafetz, M. D., & Biondolillo, A. M. (2013). Feigning a severe impairment profile. *Archives of Clinical Neuropsychology, 28,* 205–212.

Chafetz, M. D., & Dufrene, M. (2014). Malingering-by-proxy: Need for child protection and guidance for reporting. *Child Abuse and Neglect, 38,* 1755–1765.

Chafetz, M. D., & Prentkowski, E. (2011). A case of malingering by proxy in a Social Security disability psychological consultative examination. *Applied Neuropsychology, 18,* 143–149.

Chafetz, M. D., Williams, M. A., Ben-Porath, Y. S., Bianchini, K. J., Boone, K. B., Kirkwood, M. W., ... Ord, J. S. (2015). Official position of the American Academy of Clinical Neuropsychology Social Security Administration policy on validity testing: Guidance and recommendations for change. *Clinical Neuropsychologist, 29,* 723–740.

Cicerone, K., & Kalmar, K. (1995). Persistent post-concussive syndrome: Structure of subjective complaints after mild traumatic brain injury. *Journal of Head Trauma Rehabilitation, 10,* 1–17.

Cifu, D. X. (Ed.). (2016). *Braddom's physical medicine and rehabilitation* (5th ed.). Philadelphia, PA: Elsevier.

Clerico, C. M. (1989). Occupational therapy and epilepsy. *Occupational Therapy in Health Care, 6,* 41–74.

Cochrane, H. J., Baker, G. A., & Meudell, P. R. (1998). Simulating a memory impairment: can amnesics implicitly outperform simulators? *British Journal of Clinical Psychology, 37*(Pt 1), 31–48.

Cohen, R. J., Swerdlik, M. E., & Smith, D. K. (1992). *Psychological testing and assessment: An introduction to tests and measurement* (2nd ed.). Mountain View, CA: Mayfield.

Connery, A. K., Peterson, R. L., Baker, D. A., & Kirkwood, M. W. (2016). The impact of pediatric neuropsychological consultation in mild traumatic brain injury: A model for providing feedback after invalid performance. *Clinical Neuropsychologist, 30,* 579–598.

Constant, E. L., Adam, S., Gillain, B., Lambert, M., Masquelier, E., & Seron, X. (2011). Cognitive deficits in patients with chronic fatigue syndrome compared to those with major depressive disorder and healthy controls. *Clinical Neurology and Neurosurgery, 113,* 295–302.

Constantinou, M., & McCaffrey, R. J. (2003). Using the TOMM for evaluating children's effort to perform optimally on neuropsychological measures. *Child Neuropsychology, 9,* 81–90.

Cooper, D. B., Nelson, L., Armistead-Jehle, P., & Bowles, A. O. (2011). Utility of the mild brain injury atypical symptoms scale as a screening measure for symptom over-reporting in Operation Enduring Freedom/Operation Iraqi Freedom service members with post-concussive complaints. *Archives of Clinical Neuropsychology, 26,* 718–727.

Costa, P. T., & McCrae, R. R. (2010). *NEO Inventories Professional Manual: NEO-PI-3, NEO-FFI-3, NEO PI-R.* Odessa, FL: Psychological Assessment Resources.

Courtney, J. C., Dinkins, J. P., Allen, L. M., 3rd, & Kuroski, K. (2003). Age related effects in children taking the Computerized Assessment of Response Bias and Word Memory Test. *Child Neuropsychology, 9,* 109–116.

Creed, F. H., & Barsky, A. (2004). A systematic review of the epidemiology of somatisation disorder and hypochondriasis. *Journal of Psychosomatic Research, 56,* 391–408.

Cruickshank, T. M., Thompson, J. A., Dominguez, D. J. F., Reyes, A. P., Bynevelt, M., Georgiou-Karistianis, N., ... Ziman, M. R. (2015). The effect of multidisciplinary rehabilitation on brain structure and cognition in Huntington's disease: An exploratory study. *Brain and Behavior, 5,* 1–10.

Danzl, M. M., Etter, N. M., Andreatta, R. D., & Kitzman, P. H. (2012). Facilitating neurorehabilitation through principles of engagement. *Journal of Allied Health, 41,* 35–41.

Davis, J. J. (2014). Further consideration of Advanced Clinical Solutions Word Choice: Comparison to the Recognition Memory Test-words and classification accuracy in a clinical sample. *Clinical Neuropsychologist, 28,* 1278–1294.

Dawes, R. M., Faust, D., & Meehl, P. E. (1989). Clinical versus actuarial judgment. *Science, 243,* 1668–1674.

Dean, A. C., Victor, T. L., Boone, K. B., Philpott, L. M., & Hess, R. A. (2009). Dementia and effort test performance. *The Clinical Neuropsychologist, 23,* 133–152.

Delis, D. C., & Wetter, S. R. (2007). Cogniform disorder and cogniform condition: Proposed diagnoses for excessive cognitive symptoms. *Archives of Clinical Neuropsychology, 22,* 589–604.

Demakis, G. J., Gervais, R. O., & Rohling, M. L. (2008). The effect of failure on cognitive and psychological symptom validity tests in litigants with symptoms of post-traumatic stress disorder. *Clinical Neuropsychologist, 22,* 879–895.

Denning, J. H. (2012). The efficiency and accuracy of the Test of Memory Malingering trial 1, errors on the first 10 items of the test of memory malingering, and five embedded measures in predicting invalid test performance. *Archives of Clinical Neuropsychology, 27,* 417–432.

Deright, J., & Carone, D. A. (2015). Assessment of effort in children: A systematic review. *Child Neuropsychology, 21,* 1–24.

DeRight, J., & Jorgensen, R. S. (2015). I just want my research credit: Frequency of suboptimal effort in a non-clinical healthy undergraduate sample. *Clinical Neuropsychologist, 29,* 101–117.

Dersh, J., Gatchel, R. J., & Polatin, P. (2001). Chronic spinal disorders and psychopathology: Research findings and theoretical considerations. *Spine Journal, 1,* 88–94.

DiFazio, M., Silverberg, N. D., Kirkwood, M. W., Bernier, R., & Iverson, G. L. (2015). Prolonged activity restriction after concussion: Are we worsening outcomes?, *Clinical Pediatrics, 55*, 443–451.

Disorbio, J. M., & Bruns, D. (2002). *Brief Battery for Health Improvement-2 manual*. Minneapolis, MN: Pearson.

Donders, J. (2005). Performance on the Test of Memory Malingering in a mixed pediatric sample. *Child Neuropsychology, 11*, 221–227.

Donders, J., & Kirkwood, M. W. (2013). Symptom validity assessment with special populations. In D. A. Carone & S. S. Bush (Eds.), *Mild traumatic brain injury: Symptom validity assessment and malingering* (pp. 399–410). New York: Springer Publishing Company.

Dragon, W. R., Ben-Porath, Y. S., & Handel, R. W. (2012). Examining the impact of unscorable item responses on the validity and interpretability of MMPI-2/MMPI-2-RF restructured clinical (RC) scale scores. *Assessment, 19*, 101–113.

Drane, D. L., Williamson, D. J., Stroup, E. S., Holmes, M. D., Jung, M., Koerner, E., . . . Miller, J. W. (2006). Cognitive impairment is not equal in patients with epileptic and psychogenic nonepileptic seizures. *Epilepsia, 47*, 1879–1886.

Duff, K., Spering, C. C., O'Bryant, S. E., Beglinger, L. J., Moser, D. J., Bayless, J. D., . . . Scott, J. G. (2011). The RBANS Effort Index: Base rates in geriatric samples. *Applied Neuropsychology, 18*, 11–17.

Dunham, K. J., Shadia, S., Sofkoa, C. A., Denney, R. L., & Calloway, J. (2014). Comparison of the Repeatable Battery for the Assessment of Neuropsychological Status effort scale and effort index in a dementia sample. *Archives of Clinical Neuropsychology, 29*, 633–641.

Eastwood, S., & Bisson, J. I. (2008). Management of factitious disorders: A systematic review. *Psychotherapy and Psychosomatics, 77*, 209–218.

Echemendia, R. J., & Cantu, R. C. (2003). Return to play following sports-related mild traumatic brain injury: the role for neuropsychology. *Applied Neuropsychology, 10*, 48–55.

Eichstaedt, K. E., Clifton, W. E., Vale, F. L., Benbadis, S. R., Bozorg, A. M., Rodgers-Neame, N. T., & Schoenberg, M. R. (2014). Sensitivity of Green's Word Memory Test genuine memory impairment profile to temporal pathology: A study in patients with temporal lobe epilepsy. *Clinical Neuropsychologist, 28*, 941–953.

Eisendrath, S. J. (1989). Factitious physical disorders: Treatment without confrontation. *Psychosomatics, 30*, 383–387.

Elliott, R., McKinley, S., Fien, M., & Elliott, D. (2016). Posttraumatic stress symptoms in intensive care patients: An exploration of associated factors. *Rehabilitation Psychology, 61*, 141–150.

Erdodi, L. A., Kirsch, N. L., Lajiness-O'Neill, R., Vingilis, E., & Medoff, B. (2014). Comparing the Recognition Memory Test and the Word Choice Test in a mixed clinical sample: Are they equivalent? *Psychological Injury and Law, 7*, 255–263.

Erdodi, L. A., Tyson, B. T., Abeare, C. A., Zuccato, B. G., Rai, J. K., Seke, K. R., . . . Roth, R. M. (2017). Utility of critical items within the Recognition Memory Test and Word Choice Test. *Applied Neuropsychology: Adult* (published online).

Erdodi, L. A., Tyson, B. T., Shahein, A. G., Lichtenstein, J. D., Abeare, C. A., Pelletier, C. L., . . . Roth, R. M. (2017). The power of timing: Adding a time-to-completion cutoff to the Word Choice Test and Recognition Memory Test improves classification accuracy. *Journal of Clinical and Experimental Neuropsychology, 39*, 369–383.

Etherton, J. L. (2014). Diagnosing malingering in chronic pain. *Psychological Injury and Law, 7,* 362–369.

Fadil, H., Kelley, R. E., & Gonzalez-Toledo, E. (2007). Differential diagnosis of multiple sclerosis. *International Review of Neurobiology, 79,* 393–422.

Feinstein, A., Ouchterlony, D., Somerville, J., & Jardine, A. (2001). The effects of litigation on symptom expression: A prospective study following mild traumatic brain injury. *Medical Science and the Law, 41,* 116–121.

Fenton, J. J., Jerant, A. F., Bertakis, K. D., & Franks, P. (2012). The cost of satisfaction: A national study of patient satisfaction, health care utilization, expenditures, and mortality. *Archives of Internal Medicine, 172,* 405–411.

Fischer, J. S., Rudick, R. A., Cutter, G. R., & Reingold, S. C. (1999). The Multiple Sclerosis Functional Composite Measure (MSFC): An integrated approach to MS clinical outcome assessment. National MS Society Clinical Outcomes Assessment Task Force. *Multiple Sclerosis, 5,* 244–250.

Fishbain, D. A., Cutler, R., Rosomoff, H. L., & Rosomoff, R. S. (1999). Chronic pain disability exaggeration/malingering and submaximal effort research. *Clinical Journal of Pain, 15,* 244–274.

Fleming, A., & Rucas, K. (2015). Welcoming a paradigm shift in occupational therapy: Symptom validity measures and cognitive assessment. *Applied Neuropsychology: Adult, 22,* 23–31.

Frank, R. G., Rosenthal, M., & Caplan, B. (Eds.). (2010). *Handbook of rehabilitation psychology* (2nd ed.). Washington, DC: American Psychological Association.

Fukuda, K., Straus, S. E., Hickie, I., Sharpe, M. C., Dobbins, J. G., & Komaroff, A. (1994). The chronic fatigue syndrome: A comprehensive approach to its definition and study. International Chronic Fatigue Syndrome Study Group. *Annals of Internal Medicine, 121,* 953–959.

Freeman, T., Powell, M., & Kimbrell, T. (2008). Measuring symptom exaggeration in Veterans with chronic posttraumatic stress disorder. *Psychiatry Research, 158,* 347–380.

Garberding, V. (2009). Mutual trust: The key to successful assessment and treatment. *Topics in Stroke Rehabilitation, 16,* 431–436.

Gatchel, R. J., & Gardea, M. A. (1999). Psychosocial issues: Their importance in predicting disability, response to treatment, and search for compensation. *Neurologic Clinics, 17,* 149–166.

Gervais, R. O., Ben-Porath, Y. S., Wygant, D. B., & Green, P. (2007). Development and validation of a Response Bias Scale (RBS) for the MMPI-2. *Assessment, 14,* 196–208.

Gervais, R. O., Green, P., Allen, L. M., & Iverson, G. L. (2001). Effects of coaching on symptom validity testing in chronic pain patients presenting for disability assessment. *Journal of Forensic Neuropsychology, 2,* 1–19.

Gervais, R. O., Rohling, M. L., Green, P., & Ford, W. (2004). A comparison of WMT, CARB, and TOMM failure rates in non-head injury disability claimants. *Archives of Clinical Neuropsychology, 19,* 475–487.

Gervais, R. O., Russell, A. S., Green, P., Allen, L. M., Ferrari, R., & Pieschl, S. D. (2001b). Effort testing in patients with fibromyalgia and disability incentives. *Journal of Rheumatology, 28,* 1892–1899.

Gioia, G., Isquith, P. K., Guy, S. C., & Kenworthy, L. (2015). *Behavior Rating Inventory of Executive Function, Second Edition.* Lutz, FL: PAR.

Gittelman, D. K. (1998). Malingered dementia associated with battered women's syndrome. *Psychosomatics, 39,* 449–452.

Goldberg, H. E., Back-Madruga, C., & Boone, K. B. (2007). The impact of psychiatric disorders on cognitive symptom validity. In K. B. Boone (Ed.), *Assessment of feigned cognitive impairment: A neuropsychological perspective* (pp. 281–309). New York, NY: Guilford.

Gorissen, M., Sanz, J. C., & Schmand, B. (2005). Effort and cognition in schizophrenia patients. *Schizophrenia Research, 78*, 199–208.

Gouvier, W. D., Cubic, B., Jones, G., Brantley, P., & Cutlip, Q. (1992). Postconcussion symptoms and daily stress in normal and head-injured college populations. *Archives of Clinical Neuropsychology, 7*, 193–211.

Grace, J., & Malloy, P. F. (2001). *Frontal Systems Behavior Scale: Professional manual*. Lutz, FL: Psychological Assessment Resources, Inc.

Green, D., & Rosenfeld, B. (2011). Evaluating the gold standard: A review and meta-analysis of the Structured Interview of Reported Symptoms. *Psychological Assessment, 23*, 95–107.

Green, P. (2003). *Green's Word Memory Test for Windows: User's manual*. Edmonton, Alberta, Canada: Green's Publishing.

Green, P. (2004a). *Green's Medical Symptom Validity Test (MSVT) for Microsoft Windows (user manual)*. Edmonton, Alberta, Canada: Green's Publishing.

Green, P. (2004b). *Green's Memory Complaints Inventory (MCI)*. Edmonton, Alberta, Canada: Green's Publishing.

Green, P. (2007). The pervasive influence of effort on neuropsychological tests. *Physical Medicine and Rehabilitation Clinics of North America, 18*, 43–68, vi.

Green, P. (2008). *Green's Non-Verbal Medical Symptom Validity Test (NV-MSVT) for Microsoft Windows: User's Manual 1.0*. Edmonton, Alberta, Canada: Green's Publishing.

Green, P. (2009). *The Advanced Interpretation program for the WMT, MSVT, NV-MSVT and MCI*. Edmonton, Alberta, Canada: Green's Publishing.

Green, P., Allen, L. M., & Astner, K. (1996). *The Word Memory Test: A user's guide to the oral and computer-administered forms*. Edmonton, Alberta, Canada: Green's Publishing.

Green, P., Iverson, G. L., & Allen, L. (1999). Detecting malingering in head injury litigation with the Word Memory Test. *Brain Injury, 13*, 813–819.

Green, P., & Merten, T. (2013). Noncredible explanations of noncredible performance on symptom validity tests. In D. A. Carone & S. Bush (Eds.), *Mild traumatic brain injury: Symptom validity assessment and malingering* (pp. 73–99). New York, NY: Springer.

Green, P., Rohling, M. L., Lees-Haley, P. R., & Allen, L. M., 3rd. (2001). Effort has a greater effect on test scores than severe brain injury in compensation claimants. *Brain Injury, 15*, 1045–1060.

Gregory, R. J. (2014). *Psychological testing: History, principles, and applications* (7th ed.). Upper Saddle River, NJ: Pearson.

Greiffenstein, M. F. (2009). Clinical myths of forensic neuropsychology. *Clinical Neuropsychologist, 23*, 286–296.

Greiffenstein, M. F., Baker, W. J., & Gola, T. (1994). Validation of malingered amnesic measures in a large clinical sample. *Psychological Assessment, 6*, 218–224.

Greiffenstein, M. F., Baker, W. J., & Gola, T. (1996). Motor dysfunction profiles in traumatic brain injury and postconcussion syndrome. *Journal of the International Neuropsychological Society, 2*, 477–485.

Greiffenstein, M. F., Baker, W. J., & Johnson-Greene, D. (2002). Actual versus self-reported scholastic achievement of litigating postconcussion and severe closed head injury claimants. *Psychological Assessment, 14*, 202–208.

Greve, K. W., & Bianchini, K. J. (2004). Setting empirical cut-offs on psychometric indicators of negative response bias: A methodological commentary with recommendations. *Archives of Clinical Neuropsychology, 19,* 533–541.

Greve, K. W., Bianchini, K. J., Etherton, J. L., Meyers, J. E., Curtis, K. L., & Ord, J. S. (2010). The Reliable Digit Span test in chronic pain: Classification accuracy in detecting malingered pain-related disability. *Clinical Neuropsychologist, 24,* 137–152.

Greve, K. W., Bianchini, K. J., Etherton, J. L., Ord, J. S., & Curtis, K. L. (2009). Detecting malingered pain-related disability: Classification accuracy of the Portland Digit Recognition Test. *Clinical Neuropsychologist, 23,* 850–869.

Greve, K. W., Bianchini, K. J., Love, J. M., Brennan, A., & Heinly, M. T. (2006). Sensitivity and specificity of MMPI-2 validity scales and indicators to malingered neurocognitive dysfunction in traumatic brain injury. *Clinical Neuropsychologist, 20,* 491–512.

Greve, K. W., Etherton, J. L., Ord, J., Bianchini, K. J., & Curtis, K. (2009). Detecting malingered pain-related disability: Classification accuracy of the Test of Memory Malingering. *Clinical Neuropsychologist, 23,* 1250–1271.

Greve, K. W., Ord, J., Bianchini, K. J., Etherton, J. L., & Curtis, K. (2009). Prevalence of malingering in patients with chronic pain referred for psychologic evaluation in a medico-legal context. *Archives of Physical Medicine and Rehabilitation, 90,* 1117–1126.

Gross, D. P., & Battie, M. C. (2005). Factors influencing results of functional capacity evaluations in workers' compensation claimants with low back pain. *Physical Therapy, 85,* 315–322.

Grote, C. L., Kooker, E. K., Garron, D. C., Nyenhuis, D. L., Smith, C. A., & Mattingly, M. L. (2000). Performance of compensation seeking and non-compensation seeking samples on the Victoria Symptom Validity Test: Cross-validation and extension of a standardization study. *Journal of Clinical and Experimental Neuropsychology, 22,* 709–719.

Guilmette, T. J. (2013). The role of clinical judgment in symptom validity assessment. In D. A. Carone & S. S. Bush (Eds.), *Mild traumatic brain injury: Symptom validity assessment and malingering* (pp. 31–43). New York, NY: Springer.

Gunstad, J., & Suhr, J. A. (2001). "Expectation as etiology" versus "the good old days": postconcussion syndrome symptom reporting in athletes, headache sufferers, and depressed individuals. *Journal of the International Neuropsychological Society, 7,* 323–333.

Haber, A. H., & Fichtenberg, N. L. (2006). Replication of the Test of Memory Malingering (TOMM) in a traumatic brain injury and head trauma sample. *Clinical Neuropsychologist, 20,* 524–532.

Hanley, J. R., Baker, G. A., & Ledson, S. (1999). Detecting the faking of amnesia: a comparison of the effectiveness of three different techniques for distinguishing simulators from patients with amnesia. *Journal of Clinical and Experimental Neuropsychology, 21,* 59–69.

Harman, K., Macrae, M., Vallis, M., & Bassett, R. (2014). Working with people to make changes: A behavioural change approach used in chronic low back pain rehabilitation. *Physiotherapy Canada, 66,* 82–90.

Harrison, A. G., Flaro, L., & Armstrong, I. (2015). Rates of effort test failure in children with ADHD: An exploratory study. *Applied Neuropsychology: Child, 4,* 197–210.

Hartman, D. E. (2002). The unexamined lie is a lie worth fibbing: Neuropsychological testing and the Word Memory Test. *Archives of Clinical Neuropsychology, 17,* 709–714.

Hathaway, S. R., & McKinley, J. C. (1943). *Manual for administering and scoring the MMPI.* Minneapolis: University of Minnesota Press.

Heilbronner, R. L., Sweet, J. J., Morgan, J. E., Larrabee, G. J., Millis, S. R., & Conference Participants. (2009). American Academy of Clinical Neuropsychology Consensus Conference Statement on the neuropsychological assessment of effort, response bias, and malingering. *Clinical Neuropsychologist, 23*, 1093–1129.

Heinly, M. T., Greve, K. W., Bianchini, K. J., Love, J. M., & Brennan, A. (2005). WAIS digit span-based indicators of malingered neurocognitive dysfunction: Classification accuracy in traumatic brain injury. *Assessment, 12*, 429–444.

Henry, M., Merten, T., Wolf, S. A., & Harth, S. (2010). Nonverbal Medical Symptom Validity Test performance of elderly healthy adults and clinical neurology patients. *Journal of Clinical and Experimental Neuropsychology, 32*, 19–27.

Henry, G. K., Heilbronner, R. L., Algina, J., & Kaya, Y. (2013). Derivation of the MMPI-2-RF Henry-Heilbronner Index-r (HHI-r) scale. *Clinical Neuropsychologist, 27*, 509–515.

Henry, G. K., Heilbronner, R. L., Mittenberg, W., & Enders, C. (2006). The Henry-Heilbronner Index: A 15-item empirically derived MMPI-2 subscale for identifying probable malingering in personal injury litigants and disability claimants. *Clinical Neuropsychologist, 20*, 786–797.

Hibbard, M. R., & Cox, D. R. (2010). Competencies of a rehabilitation psychologist. In R. G. Frank, M. Rosenthal, & B. Caplan (Eds.), *Handbook of rehabilitation psychology* (pp. 467–475). Washington, DC: American Psychological Association.

Hilsabeck, R. C., Gordon, S. N., Hietpas-Wilson, T., & Zartman, A. L. (2011). Use of Trial 1 of the Test of Memory Malingering (TOMM) as a screening measure of effort: Suggested discontinuation rules. *Clinical Neuropsychologist, 25*, 1228–1238.

Hiller, W., Rief, W., & Brahler, E. (2006). Somatization in the population: from mild bodily misperceptions to disabling symptoms. *Social Psychiatry and Psychiatric Epidemiology, 41*, 704–712.

Hoffmaster, E., Lech, R., & Niebuhr, B. R. (1993). Consistency of sincere and feigned grip exertions with repeated testing. *Journal of Occupational Medicine, 35*, 788–794.

Hogan, T. P. (2015). *Psychological testing: A practical introduction* (3rd ed.). Hoboken, NJ: Wiley.

Holdnack, J. A., & Drozdick, L. W. (2008). *An introduction to Advanced Clinical Solutions for the WAIS-IV and WMS-IV (ACS)*. Retrieved October 27, 2016, from http://www.pearsonclinical.com/psychology/products/100000616/advanced-clinical-solutions-for-the-wais-iv-and-wms-iv-acs.html#tab-resources

Hook, J. N., Marquine, M. J., & Hoelzle, J. B. (2009). Repeatable Battery for the Assessment of Neuropsychological Status effort index performance in a medically ill geriatric sample. *Archives of Clinical Neuropsychology, 24*, 231–235.

Horner, M. D., VanKirk, K. K., Dismuke, C. E., Turner, T. H., & Muzzy, W. (2014). Inadequate effort on neuropsychological evaluation is associated with increased healthcare utilization. *Clinical Neuropsychologist, 28*, 703–713.

Hoskins, L. L., Binder, L. M., Chaytor, N. S., Williamson, D. J., & Drane, D. L. (2010). Comparison of oral and computerized versions of the word memory test. *Archives of Clinical Neuropsychology, 25*, 591–600.

Howe, L. L., Anderson, A. M., Kaufman, D. A., Sachs, B. C., & Loring, D. W. (2007). Characterization of the Medical Symptom Validity Test in evaluation of clinically referred memory disorders clinic patients. *Archives of Clinical Neuropsychology, 22*, 753–761.

Howe, L. L., & Loring, D. W. (2009). Classification accuracy and predictive ability of the Medical Symptom Validity Test's dementia profile and general memory impairment profile. *The Clinical Neuropsychologist, 23,* 329–342.

Huet, E. (2012). Ayres to be retried on molest charges. Retrieved 03/02/2017, from http://www.sfgate.com/crime/article/Ayres-to-be-retried-on-molest-charges-4001692.php

Hutchinson, B. D., Navin, P., Marom, E. M., Truong, M. T., & Bruzzi, J. F. (2015). Overdiagnosis of pulmonary embolism by pulmonary CT angiography. *AJR: American Journal of Roentgenology, 205,* 271–277.

Incesu, A. I. (2013). Tests for malingering in ophthalmology. *International Journal of Ophthalmology, 6,* 708–717.

Iverson, G. L. (2007). Assessing for exaggeration, poor effort, and malingering in neuropsychological assessment. In A. M. Horton & D. Wedding (Eds.), *The neuropsychology handbook.* New York, NY: Springer.

Iverson, G. L., Franzen, M. D., & McCracken, L. M. (1991). Evaluation of a standardized instrument for the detection of malingered memory deficits. *Law and Human Behavior, 15,* 667–676.

Iverson, G. L., King, R. J., Scott, J. G., & Adams, R. L. (2001). Cognitive complaints in litigating patients with head injuries or chronic pain. *Journal of Forensic Neuropsychology, 2,* 19–30.

Iverson, G. L., Le Page, J., Koehler, B. E., Shojania, K., & Badii, M. (2007). Test of Memory Malingering Scores are not affected by chronic pain or depression in patients with fibromyalgia. *Clinical Psychologist, 21,* 532–546.

Iverson, G. L., & McCracken, L. M. (1997). "Postconcussive" symptoms in persons with chronic pain. *Brain Injury, 11,* 783–790.

Johnson, S. K. (2008). *Medically unexplained illness: Gender and biopsychosocial implications.* Washington, DC: APA Books.

Johnson-Greene, D., Brooks, L., & Ference, T. (2013). Relationship between performance validity testing, disability status, and somatic complaints in patients with fibromyalgia. *Clinical Neuropsychologist, 27,* 148–158.

Jones, A. (2013). Victoria Symptom Validity Test: Cutoff scores for psychometrically defined malingering groups in a military sample. *Clinical Neuropsychologist, 27,* 1373–1394.

Jones, E., Pike, J., Marshall, T., & Ye, X. (2016). Quantifying the relationship between increased disability and health care resource utilization, quality of life, work productivity, health care costs in patients with multiple sclerosis in the US. *BMC Health Services Research, 16,* 294.

Kaplan, R. M., & Saccuzzo, D. P. (2013). *Psychological testing: Principles, applications, and issues.* Belmont, CA: Wadsworth Cengage Learning.

Kapur, N. (1994). The coin-in-the-hand test: a new "bed-side" test for the detection of malingering in patients with suspected memory disorder. *Journal of Neurology, Neurosurgery and Psychiatry, 57,* 385–386.

Kaufman, D. M. (2006). Functional psychogenic deficits. In *Clinical Neurology for Psychiatrists* (6th ed., pp. 19–26). Philadelphia, PA: Saunders Elsevier.

Keary, T. A., Frazier, T. W., Belzile, C. J., Chapin, J. S., Naugle, R. I., Najm, I. M., & Busch, R. M. (2013). Working memory and intelligence are associated with Victoria Symptom Validity Test hard item performance in patients with intractable epilepsy. *Journal of the International Neuropsychological Society, 19,* 314–323.

Kelly, P. J., Baker, G. A., van den Broek, M. D., Jackson, H., & Humphries, G. (2005). The detection of malingering in memory performance: the sensitivity and specificity of four measures in a UK population. *British Journal of Clinical Psychology, 44*, 333–341.

Kennedy, P. (Ed.). (2012). *The Oxford handbook of rehabilitation psychology.* New York, NY: Oxford University Press.

Khan, F., & Amatya, B. (2016). Rehabilitation in multiple sclerosis: A systematic review of systematic reviews. *Archives of Physical Medicine and Rehabilitation.*

King, P. M., Tuckwell, N., & Barrett, T. E. (1998). A critical review of functional capacity evaluations. *Physical Therapy, 78,* 852–866.

Kirk, J. W., Harris, B., Hutaff-Lee, C. F., Koelemay, S. W., Dinkins, J. P., & Kirkwood, M. W. (2011). Performance on the Test of Memory Malingering (TOMM) among a large clinic-referred pediatric sample. *Child Neuropsychology, 17,* 242–254.

Kirkwood, M. W. (2015). Review of pediatric performance and symptom validity tests. In M. W. Kirkwood (Ed.), *Validity testing in child and adolescent assessment: Evaluating exaggeration, feigning, and non-credible effort* (pp. 79–106). New York, NY: Guilford.

Kirkwood, M. W., Kirk, J. W., Blaha, R. Z., & Wilson, P. (2010). Noncredible effort during pediatric neuropsychological exam: A case series and literature review. *Child Neuropsychology, 16,* 604–618.

Knapp, S. J., VandeCreek, L. D., & Fingerhut, R. (2017). *Practical ethics for psychologists: A positive approach* (3rd ed.). Washington, DC: American Psychological Association.

Knoll, J., & Resnick, P. J. (2006). The detection of malingered post-traumatic stress disorder. *Psychiatric Clinics of North America, 29,* 629–647.

Korakas, N., & Tsolaki, M. (2016). Cognitive Impairment in Multiple Sclerosis: A review of neuropsychological assessments. *Cognitive and Behavioral Neurology, 29,* 55–67.

Kozora, E., Arciniegas, D. B., Zhang, L., & West, S. (2007). Neuropsychological patterns in systemic lupus erythematosus patients with depression. *Arthritis Research & Therapy, 9,* R48.

Kurtzke, J. F. (1983). Rating neurologic impairment in multiple sclerosis: An expanded disability status scale (EDSS). *Neurology, 33,* 1444–1452.

Lamberty, G. J. (2008). *Understanding somatization in the practice of clinical neuropsychology.* New York, NY: Oxford University Press.

Lange, R. T., Brickell, T. A., Lippa, S. M., & French, L. M. (2015). Clinical utility of the Neurobehavioral Status Exam validity scales to screen for symptom exaggeration following traumatic brain injury. *Journal of Clinical and Experimental Neuropsychology, 37,* 853–862.

Langhorne, P., Bernhardt, J., & Kwakkel, G. (2011). Stroke rehabilitation. *Lancet, 377,* 1693–1702.

Larrabee, G. J. (2003). Exaggerated MMPI-2 symptom report in personal injury litigants with malingered neurocognitive deficit. *Archives of Clinical Neuropsychology, 18,* 673–686.

Larrabee, G. (2005a). Assessment of malingering. In G. Larrabee (Ed.), *Forensic neuropsychology: A scientific approach* (pp. 115–158). New York, NY: Oxford University Press.

Larrabee, G. (Ed.). (2005b). *Forensic neuropsychology: A scientific approach.* New York, NY: Oxford University Press.

Larrabee, G. J. (2007). Evaluation of exaggerated health and injury symptomatology. In G. J. Larrabee (Ed.), *Assessment of malingered neuropsychological deficits* (pp. 264–286). New York, NY: Oxford University Press.

Larrabee, G. J. (2012). Performance validity and symptom validity in neuropsychological assessment. *Journal of the International Neuropsychological Society, 18,* 625–630.

Larson, E., Zollman, F., Kondiles, B., & Starr, C. (2013). Memory deficits, postconcussive complaints, and posttraumatic stress disorder in a volunteer sample of veterans. *Rehabilitation Psychology, 58*, 245–252.

LeBourgeois, H. (2007). Malingering: Key points in assessment. *Psychiatric Times, 24*, 21–32.

Lechner, D. E., Bradbury, S. F., & Bradley, L. A. (1998). Detecting sincerity of effort: A summary of methods and approaches. *Physical Therapy, 78*, 867–888.

Lees-Haley, P. R., & Brown, R. S. (1993). Neuropsychological complaint base rates of 170 personal injury claimants. *Archives of Clinical Neuropsychology, 8*, 203–209.

Lees-Haley, P. R., English, L. T., & Glenn, W. J. (1991). A fake bad scale on the MMPI-2 for personal injury claimants. *Psychological Reports, 68*, 203–210.

Lees-Haley, P. R., Fox, D. D., & Courtney, J. C. (2001). A comparison of complaints by mild brain injury claimants and other claimants describing subjective experiences immediately following their injury. *Archives of Clinical Neuropsychology, 16*, 689–695.

Lempert, T., Brandt, T., Dieterich, M., & Huppert, D. (1991). How to identify psychogenic disorders of stance and gait: A video study in 37 patients. *Journal of Neurology, 238*, 140–146.

Lemstra, M., Olszynski, W. P., & Enright, W. (2004). The sensitivity and specificity of functional capacity evaluations in determining maximal effort: A randomized trial. *Spine (Phila Pa 1976), 29*, 953–959.

Lew, H. L., Otis, J. D., Tun, C., Kerns, R. D., Clark, M. E., & Cifu, D. X. (2009). Prevalence of chronic pain, posttraumatic stress disorder, and persistent postconcussive symptoms in OIF/OEF veterans: Polytrauma clinical triad. *Journal of Rehabilitation Research and Development, 46*, 697–702.

Lezak, M. D., Howieson, D. B., Bigler, E. D., & Tranel, D. (2012). *Neuropsychological assessment* (5th ed.). New York, NY: Oxford University Press.

Linton, S. J. (2000). A review of psychological risk factors in back and neck pain. *Spine, 25*, 1148–1156.

Locke, D. E., Smigielski, J. S., Powell, M. R., & Stevens, S. R. (2008). Effort issues in post-acute outpatient acquired brain injury rehabilitation seekers. *NeuroRehabilitation, 23*, 273–281.

Loring, D. W., Lee, G. P., & Meador, K. J. (2005). Victoria Symptom Validity Test performance in non-litigating epilepsy surgery candidates. *Journal of Clinical and Experimental Neuropsychology, 27*, 610–617.

Loring, D. W., Goldstein, F. C., Chen, C., Drane, D. L., Lah, J. J., Zhao, L., & Larrabee, G. J. (2016). False-Positive Error Rates for Reliable Digit Span and Auditory Verbal Learning Test Performance Validity Measures in Amnestic Mild Cognitive Impairment and Early Alzheimer Disease. *Archives of Clinical Neuropsychology, 31*, 313–331.

Lu, P. H., & Boone, K. B. (2002). Suspect cognitive symptoms in a 9-year-old child: Malingering by proxy? *Clinical Neuropsychologist, 16*, 90–96.

Lynch, W. J. (2004). Determination of effort level, exaggeration, and malingering in neurocognitive assessment. *Journal of Head Trauma Rehabilitation, 19*, 277–283.

MacAllister, W. S., Nakhutina, L., Bender, H. A., Karantzoulis, S., & Carlson, C. (2009). Assessing effort during neuropsychological evaluation with the TOMM in children and adolescents with epilepsy. *Child Neuropsychology, 15*, 521–531.

Macciocchi, S. N., Seel, R. T., Alderson, A., & Godsall, R. (2006). Victoria Symptom Validity Test performance in acute severe traumatic brain injury: Implications for test interpretation. *Archives of Clinical Neuropsychology, 21*, 395–404.

Martin, P. K., Schroeder, R. W., & Odland, A. P. (2015). Neuropsychologists' validity testing beliefs and practices: A survey of North American professionals. *Clinical Neuropsychologist, 29,* 741–776.

Mason, A. M., Cardell, R., & Armstrong, M. (2014). Malingering psychosis: Guidelines for assessment and management. *Perspectives in Psychiatric Care, 50,* 51–57.

Mathias, C. W., Greve, K. W., Bianchini, K. J., Houston, R. J., & Crouch, J. A. (2002). Detecting malingered neurocognitive dysfunction using the reliable digit span in traumatic brain injury. *Assessment, 9,* 301–308.

Mazur-Mosiewicz, A., Carlson, H. L., Hartwick, C., Dykeman, J., Lenders, T., Brooks, B. L., & Wiebe, S. (2015). Effectiveness of cognitive rehabilitation following epilepsy surgery: Current state of knowledge. *Epilepsia, 56,* 735–744.

McCann, J. T. (1998). *Malingering and Decepption in Adolescents: Assessing Credibility in Clinical and Forensic Settings.* Washington, D.C.: American Psychological Association.

McCaffrey, R. J., & Lynch, J. K. (2009). Malingering following documented brain injury: Neuropsychological evaluation of children in a forensic setting. In J. E. Morgan & J. J. Sweet (Eds.), *Neuropsychology of malingering casebook* (pp. 377–385). New York, NY: Psychology Press.

McCracken, L. M., & Thompson, M. (2012). Neuropsychological aspects of chronic pain. In S. S. Bush & G. L. Iverson (Eds.), *Neuropsychological assessment of work-related injuries* (pp. 243–262). New York, NY: Guilford Press.

McCrea, M. (2008). *Mild traumatic brain injury and postconcussion syndrome: The new evidence base for diagnosis and treatment.* New York, NY: Oxford University Press.

McCrea, M., Guskiewicz, K., Randolph, C., Barr, W. B., Hammeke, T. A., Marshall, S. W., & Kelly, J. P. (2009). Effects of a symptom-free waiting period on clinical outcome and risk of reinjury after sport-related concussion. *Neurosurgery, 65,* 876–882; discussion 882–873.

McCullumsmith, C. B., & Ford, C. V. (2011). Simulated illness: The factitious disorders and malingering. *Psychiatric Clinics of North America, 34,* 621–641.

Mehta, S. J. (2015). Patient satisfaction reporting and its implications for patient care. *AMA Journal of Ethics, 17,* 616–621.

Merten, T., & Merckelbach, H. (2013). Symptom validity testing in somatoform and dissociative disorders: A critical review. *Psychological Injury and Law, 6,* 122–137.

Meyers, J. E., Millis, S. R., & Volkert, K. (2002). A validity index for the MMPI-2. *Archives of Clinical Neuropsychology, 17,* 157–169.

Meyers, J. E., Volbrecht, M., Axelrod, B. N., & Reinsch-Boothby, L. (2011). Embedded symptom validity tests and overall neuropsychological test performance. *Archives of Clinical Neuropsychology, 26,* 8–15.

Miller, J. B., Axelrod, B. N., Schutte, C., & Davis, J. J. (2017). Symptom and performance validity assessment in forensic neuropsychology. In S. S. Bush & A. L. Heck (Eds.), *Forensic geropsychology: Practice essentials* (pp. 67–109). Washington, DC: APA Books.

Miller, J. B., & Axelrod, B. N. (2018). Performance validity assessment: Disentangling dementia from the disinterested and disingenuous. In S. S. Bush & A. L. Heck (Eds.), *Forensic geropsychology: Practice essentials* (pp. 25–47). Washington, DC: APA Books.

Miller, L. J., & Donders, J. (2001). Subjective symptomatology after traumatic head injury. *Brain Injury, 15,* 297–304.

Millis, S. R., Rosenthal, M., Novack, T. A., Sherer, M., Nick, T. G., Kreutzer, J. S., ... Ricker, J. H. (2001). Long-term neuropsychological outcome after traumatic brain injury. *Journal of Head Trauma Rehabilitation, 16*, 343–355.

Mittenberg, W., Patton, C., Canyock, E. M., & Condit, D. C. (2002). Base rates of malingering and symptom exaggeration. *Journal of Clinical and Experimental Neuropsychology, 24*, 1094–1102.

Montoya, A., Price, B. H., Menear, M., & Lepage, M. (2006). Brain imaging and cognitive dysfunctions in Huntington's disease. *Journal of Psychiatry and Neuroscience, 31*, 21–29.

Morey, L. C. (2007). *Personality Assessment Inventory-Adolsecent: Professional manual*. Lutz, FL: Psychological Assessment Resources.

Morgan, J. E., & Ricker, J. H. (Eds.). (2008). *Textbook of clinical neuropsychology*. New York, NY: Taylor & Francis.

Morgan, J. E., & Sweet, J. J. (Eds.). (2009). *Neuropsychology of malingering casebook*. New York, NY: Taylor & Francis (Psychology Press).

Nahin, R. L. (2015). Estimates of pain prevalence and severity in adults: United States, 2012. *Journal of Pain, 16*, 769–780.

National Academy of Neuropsychology. (1998). The Houston conference on specialty education and training in clinical neuropsychology. *Archives of Clinical Neuropsychology, 13*, 160–166.

NCS Pearson Inc. (2009). *Advanced clinical solutions for the WAIS®-IV and WMS®-IV (ACS)*. San Antonio, TX: Author.

NCS Pearson Inc. (2010). *Advanced clinical solutions suboptimal effort case studies*. Retrieved October 27, 2016, from http://images.pearsonclinical.com/images/assets/ACS/471410_ACS_Suboptimal_Effort_CS_Lr_f.pdf.

Novitski, J., Steele, S., Karantzoulis, S., & Randolph, C. (2012). The Repeatable Battery for the Assessment of Neuropsychological Status effort scale. *Archives of Clinical Neuropsychology, 27*, 190–195.

Pankratz, L. (1979). Symptom validity testing and symptom retraining: Procedures for the assessment and treatment of functional sensory deficits. *Journal of Consulting and Clinical Psychology, 47*, 409–410.

Pankratz, L. (1983). A new technique for the assessment and modification of feigned memory deficit. *Perceptual and Motor Skills, 57*, 367–372.

Patel, A. T. (2001). Disability evaluation following stroke. *Physical Medicine and Rehabilitation Clinics of North America, 12*, 613–619.

Ploetz, D. M., Mazur-Mosiewicz, A., Kirkwood, M. W., Sherman, E. M., & Brooks, B. L. (2016). Performance on the Test of Memory Malingering in children with neurological conditions. *Child Neuropsychology, 22*, 133–142.

Portenoy, R. K. (1996). Opioid therapy for chronic nonmalignant pain: A review of the critical issues. *Journal of Pain and Symptom Management, 11*, 203–217.

Price, T., & Caplan, B. (2017). Cognitive screening. In M. A. Budd, S. Hough, S. T. Wegener, & W. Stiers (Eds.), *Practical psychology in medical rehabilitation* (pp. 391–396). Switzerland: Springer International.

Prigatano, G., & Morrone-Strupinsky, J. (2010). The study of anosognosia. In G. Prigatano (Ed.), *Management and rehabilitation of persons with anosognosia and impaired self-awareness*. New York, NY: Oxford University Press.

References

Putnam, S. H., & Millis, S. R. (1994). Psychological factors in the developmental and maintenance of chronic somatic and functional symptoms following mild traumatic brain injury. *Advances in Medical Psychotherapy, 7,* 1–22.

Rabin, L. A., Barr, W. B., & Burton, L. A. (2005). Assessment practices of clinical neuropsychologists in the United States and Canada: A survey of INS, NAN, and APA Division 40 members. *Archives of Clinical Neuropsychology, 20,* 33–65.

Randolph, C. (1998). *Repeatable Battery for the Assessment of Neuropsychological Status Manual.* San Antonio, TX: The Psychological Corporation.

Reich, P., & Gottfried, L. A. (1983). Factitious disorders in a teaching hospital. *Annals of Internal Medicine, 99,* 240–247.

Reid, W. H. (2003). Expert evaluation, controversial cases, and the media. *Journal of Psychiatric Practice, 9,* 388–390.

Resnick, P. J. (1997). Malingering of posttraumatic disorders. In R. Rogers (Ed.), *Clinical assessment of malingering and deception* (2nd ed., pp. 130–152). New York, NY: Guilford.

Rey, A. (1964). *L'examen clinique en psychologie.* Paris: Presses Universitaires de France.

Reynolds, C. R., & Kamphaus, R. W. (2006). *BASC-2: Behavior Assessment System for Children, Second Edition.* Upper Saddle River, NJ: Pearson Education, Inc.

Reynolds, C. R., & Horton, A. M. (Eds.). (2012). *Detection of malingering during head injury litigation* (2nd ed.). New York, NY: Springer.

Rienstra, A., Groot, P. F., Spaan, P. E., Majoie, C. B., Nederveen, A. J., Walstra, G. J., … Schmand, B. (2013). Symptom validity testing in memory clinics: Hippocampal-memory associations and relevance for diagnosing mild cognitive impairment. *Journal of Clinical and Experimental Neuropsychology, 35,* 59–70.

Rienstra, A., Klein Twennaar, M., & Schmand, B. (2013). Neuropsychological characterization of patients with the WMT dementia profile. *Archives of Clinical Neuropsychology, 28,* 463–475.

Roberts, M. D. (1997). Munchausen by proxy. *Journal of the American Academy of Child and Adolescent Psychiatry, 36,* 578–580.

Rogers, R., Gillis, J. R., Dickens, S. E., & Bagby, R. M. (1991). Standardized assessment of malingering: Validation of the SIRS. *Psychological Assessment, 3,* 89–96.

Rohling, M. L., Binder, L. M., & Langhinrichsen-Rohling, J. A. (1995). A meta-analytic review of the association between financial compensation and the experience and treatment of chronic pain. *Health Psychology, 14,* 537–547.

Rohling, M. L., & Demakis, G. J. (2010). Bowden, Shores, & Mathias (2006): Failure to replicate or just failure to notice. Does effort still account for more variance in neuropsychological test scores than TBI severity? *Clinical Neuropsychologist, 24,* 119–136.

Roor, J. J., Dandachi-FitzGerald, B., & Ponds, R. W. (2016). A case of misdiagnosis of mild cognitive impairment: The utility of symptom validity testing in an outpatient memory clinic. *Applied Neuropsychology: Adult, 23,* 172–178.

Rosen, G. M., & Powell, J. E. (2003). Use of a symptom validity test in the forensic assessment of posttraumatic stress disorder. *Journal of Anxiety Disorders, 17,* 361–367.

Ross, C. A., Pantelyat, A., Kogan, J., & Brandt, J. (2014). Determinants of functional disability in Huntington's disease: Role of cognitive and motor dysfunction. *Movement Disorders, 29,* 1351–1358.

Ross, C. A., & Tabrizi, S. J. (2011). Huntington's disease: From molecular pathogenesis to clinical treatment. *Lancet Neurology, 10,* 83–98.

Ross, T. P., Poston, A. M., Rein, P. A., Salvatore, A. N., Wills, N. L., & York, T. M. (2016). Performance invalidity base rates among healthy undergraduate research participants. *Archives of Clinical Neuropsychology, 31,* 97–104.

Roth, R. S., & Spencer, R. J. (2013). Iatrogenic risk in the management of mild traumatic brain injury among combat veterans: A case illustration and commentary. *International Journal of Physical Medicine and Rehabilitation, 1,* 1–7.

Rubenzer, S. (2009). Posttraumatic stress disorder: Assessing response style and malingering. *Psychological Injury and Law, 2,* 114–142.

Sawyer, R. J., 2nd, Testa, S. M., & Dux, M. (2016). Embedded performance validity tests within the Hopkins Verbal Learning Test—Revised and the Brief Visuospatial Memory Test—Revised. *Clinical Neuropsychologist,* 1–12.

Schagen, S., Schmand, B., de Sterke, S., & Lindeboom, J. (1997). Amsterdam Short-Term Memory test: A new procedure for the detection of feigned memory deficits. *Journal of Clinical and Experimental Neuropsychology, 19,* 43–51.

Schapmire, D., St James, J. D., Townsend, R., Stewart, T., Delheimer, S., & Focht, D. (2002). Simultaneous bilateral testing: Validation of a new protocol to detect insincere effort during grip and pinch strength testing. *Journal of Hand Therapy, 15,* 242–250.

Schatz, P., & Glatz, C. (2013). "Sandbagging" baseline test performance on ImPACT, without detection, is more difficult than it appears. *Archives of Clinical Neuropsychology, 28,* 236–244.

Schnellbacher, S., & O'Mara, H. (2016). Identifying and managing malingering and factitious disorder in the military. *Current Psychiatry Reports, 18,* 105.

Schroeder, R. W., Twumasi-Ankrah, P., Baade, L. E., & Marshall, P. S. (2012). Reliable digit span: A systematic review and cross-validation study. *Assessment, 19,* 21–30.

Sellbom, M., & Bagby, R. M. (2008). Validity of the MMPI-2-RF (Restructured Form) L-r and K-r scales in detecting underreporting in clinical and nonclinical samples. *Psychological Assessment, 20,* 370–376.

Sellbom, M., Wygant, D., & Bagby, M. (2011). Utility of the MMPI-2-RF in detecting non-credible somatic complaints. *Psychiatry Research, 197,* 295–301.

Sherer, M., Davis, L. C., Sander, A. M., Nick, T. G., Luo, C., Pastorek, N., & Hanks, R. (2015). Factors associated with Word Memory Test performance in persons with medically documented traumatic brain injury. *Clinical Neuropsychologist, 29,* 522–541.

Sherman, E. M., & Brooks, B. L. (2015). *Child and Adolscent Memory Profile (ChAMP): Professional manual.* Lutz, Florida: Psychological Assessment Resources, Inc.

Sherman, E. M., & Brooks, B. L. (2016). *Memory Validity Profile (MVP): Professional manual.* Lutz, Florida: Psychological Assessment Resources, Inc.

Sherman, E. M., & Brooks, B. L. (2017). *Multideimesnional Everyday Memory Ratings for Youth (MEMRY): Professional manual.* Lutz, Florida: Psychological Assessment Resources, Inc.

Sieck, B. C., Smith, M. M., Duff, K., Paulsen, J. S., & Beglinger, L. J. (2013). Symptom validity test performance in the Huntington Disease Clinic. *Archives of Clinical Neuropsychology, 28,* 135–143.

Silk-Eglit, G. M., Lynch, J. K., & McCaffrey, R. J. (2016). Validation of Victoria Symptom Validity Test cutoff scores among mild traumatic brain injury litigants using a known-groups design. *Archives of Clinical Neuropsychology, 31,* 231–245.

Silk-Eglit, G. M., Stenclik, J. H., Gavett, B. E., Adams, J. W., Lynch, J. K., & McCaffrey, R. J. (2014). Base rate of performance invalidity among non-clinical undergraduate research participants. *Archives of Clinical Neuropsychology, 29,* 415–421.

Silver, J. M. (2015). Invalid symptom reporting and performance: What are we missing? *NeuroRehabilitation, 36,* 463–469.

Silverberg, N.D., Iverson, G.L., & Panenka, W. (2017). Cogniphobia in mild traumatic brain injury. *Journal of Neurotrauma, 34,* 2141–2146.

Silverberg, N. D., Wertheimer, J. C., & Fichtenberg, N. L. (2007). An effort index for the Repeatable Battery for the Assessment of Neuropsychological Status (RBANS). *Clinical Neuropsychologist, 21,* 841–854.

Singhal, A., Green, P., Ashaye, K., Shankar, K., & Gill, D. (2009). High specificity of the medical symptom validity test in patients with very severe memory impairment. *Archives of Clinical Neuropsychology, 24,* 721–728.

Slick, D., Hopp, G., Strauss, E., & Thompson, G.B. (1997). *Victoria Symptom Validity Test.* Odessa, FL: Psychological Assessment Resources.

Slick, D. J., & Sherman, E. M. S. (2013). Differential diagnosis of malingering. In D. A. Carone & S. S. Bush (Eds.), *Mild traumatic brain injury: Symptom validity assessment and malingering* (pp. 57–72). New York, NY: Springer.

Slick, D., Sherman, E. M., & Iverson, G. L. (1999). Diagnostic criteria for malingered neurocognitive dysfunction: Proposed standards for clinical practice and research. *Clinical Neuropsychologist, 13,* 545–561.

Slick, D., Tan, J. E., Strauss, E., Mateer, C. A., Harnadek, M., & Sherman, E. M. (2003). Victoria Symptom Validity Test scores of patients with profound memory impairment: Nonlitigant case studies. *Clinical Neuropsychologist, 17,* 390–394.

Soble, J. R., Silva, M. A., Vanderploeg, R. D., Curtiss, G., Belanger, H. G., Donnell, A. J., & Scott, S. G. (2014). Normative Data for the Neurobehavioral Symptom Inventory (NSI) and post-concussion symptom profiles among TBI, PTSD, and nonclinical samples. *Clinical Neuropsychologist, 28,* 614–632.

Specht, U., Coban, I., Bien, C. G., & May, T. W. (2015). Risk factors for early disability pension in patients with epilepsy and vocational difficulties—Data from a specialized rehabilitation unit. *Epilepsy and Behavior, 51,* 243–248.

Speroff, T., Sinnott, P. L., Marx, B., Owen, R. R., Jackson, J. C., Greevy, R., . . . Friedman, M. J. (2012). Impact of evidence-based standardized assessment on the Disability Clinical Interview for Diagnosis of Service-Connected PTSD: A cluster-randomized trial. *Journal of Traumatic Stress, 25,* 607–615.

Stevens, A., Schneider, K., Liske, B., Hermle, L., Huber, H., & Hetzel, G. (2014). Is subnormal cognitive performance in schizophrenia due to lack of effort or cognitive impairment? *German Journal of Psychiatry, 1,* 1–9.

Stiers, W., Barisa, M., Stucky, K., Pawlowski, C., Van Tubbergen, M., Turner, A. P., . . . Caplan, B. (2015). Guidelines for competency development and measurement in rehabilitation psychology postdoctoral training. *Rehabilitation Psychology, 60,* 111–122.

Stone, J., Carson, A., & Sharpe, M. (2005). Functional symptoms and signs in neurology: Assessment and diagnosis. *Journal of Neurology, Neurosurgery and Psychiatry, 76*(Suppl 1), i2–i12.

Strauss, E., Sherman, E. M., & Spreen, O. (2006). *A compendium of neuropsychological tests: Administration, norms, and commentary* (3rd ed.). New York, NY: Oxford University Press.

Stutts, J. T., Hickey, S. E., & Kasdan, M. L. (2003). Malingering by proxy: A form of pediatric condition falsification. *Journal of Developmental and Behavioral Pediatrics, 24,* 276–278.

Suchy, Y., Chelune, G., Franchow, E. I., & Thorgusen, S. R. (2012). Confronting patients about insufficient effort: The impact on subsequent symptom validity and memory performance. *Clinical Neuropsychologist, 26,* 1296–1311.

Suhr, J. (2003). Neuropsychological impairment in fibromyalgia: Relation to depression, fatigue, and pain. *Journal of Psychosomatic Research, 55,* 321–329.

Suhr, J. A., & Gunstad, J. (2000). The effects of coaching on the sensitivity and specificity of malingering measures. *Archives of Clinical Neuropsychology, 15,* 415–424.

Suhr, J. A., & Gunstad, J. (2002). "Diagnosis threat": The effect of negative expectations on cognitive performance in head injury. *Journal of Clinical and Experimental Neuropsychology, 24,* 448–457.

Suhr, J. A., Gunstad, J., Greub, B., & Barrish, J. (2004). Exaggeration index for an expanded version of the auditory verbal learning test: Robustness to coaching. *Journal of Clinical and Experimental Neuropsychology, 26,* 416–427.

Suhr, J., & Spickard, B. (2007). Including measures of effort in neuropsychological assessment of pain- and fatigue-related medical disorders: Clinical and research implications. In K. B. Boone (Ed.), *Assessment of feigned cognitive impairment: A neuropsychological perspective* (pp. 259–280). New York, NY: Guilford.

Suhr, J., & Spickard, B. (2012). Pain-related fear is associated with cognitive task avoidance: Exploration of the cogniphobia construct in a recurrent headache sample. *The Clinical Neuropsychologist, 26,* 1128–1141.

Sung, C., Muller, V., Jones, J. E., & Chan, F. (2014). Vocational rehabilitation service patterns and employment outcomes of people with epilepsy. *Epilepsy Research, 108,* 1469–1479.

Sweet, J. J., Perry, W., Ruff, R. M., Shear, P. K., & Guidotti Breting, L. M. (2012). The Inter-Organizational Summit on Education and Training (ISET) 2010 survey on the influence of the Houston Conference training guidelines. *Clinical Neuropsychologist, 26,* 1055–1076.

Todd, D. D., Martelli, M. F., & Grayson, R. L. (1998). *The Cogniphobia Scale (C-Scale): A measure of headache impact.* Glen Allen, VA: Concussion Care Centre of Virginia.

Tolin, D. F., Steenkamp, M. M., Marx, B. P., & Litz, B. T. (2010). Detecting symptom exaggeration in combat veterans using the MMPI-2 symptom validity scales: A mixed group validation. *Psychological Assessment, 22,* 729–736.

Tombaugh, T. (1996). *Test of memory malingering.* Los Angeles: Western Psychological Services.

Trippolini, M. A., Dijkstra, P. U., Jansen, B., Oesch, P., Geertzen, J. H., & Reneman, M. F. (2014). Reliability of clinician rated physical effort determination during functional capacity evaluation in patients with chronic musculoskeletal pain. *Journal of Occupational Rehabilitation, 24,* 361–369.

van der Werf, S. P., de Vree, B., van der Meer, J. W., & Bleijenberg, G. (2002). The relations among body consciousness, somatic symptom report, and information processing speed in chronic fatigue syndrome. *Neuropsychiatry, Neuropsychology, and Behavioral Neurology, 15,* 2–9.

van der Werf, S. P., Prins, J. B., Jongen, P. H. J., van der Meer, J. W. M., & Bleijenberg, G. (2000). Abnormal neuropsychological findings are not necessarily a sign of cerebral impairment: A matched comparison between chronic fatigue syndrome and multiple sclerosis. *Neuropsychiatry, Neuropsychology, and Behavioral Neurology, 13,* 199–203.

van Impelen, A., Merckelbach, H., Jelicic, M., & Merten, T. (2014). The Structured Inventory of Malingered Symptomatology (SIMS): A systematic review and meta-analysis. *Clinical Neuropsychologist, 28,* 1336–1365.

Victor, T. V., Boone, K. B., & Kulick, A. D. (2013). Assessing non-credible sensory, motor, and executive function, and test battery performance in mild traumatic brain injury. In D. A. Carone & S. B. Bush (Eds.), *Mild traumatic brain injury: Symptom validity assessment and malingering* (pp. 269–301). New York, NY: Springer.

Victor, T. V., Kulick, A. D., & Boone, K. B. (2013). Assessing noncredible attention, processing speed, language, and visuospatial/perceptual function in mild traumatic brain injury. In D. A. Carone & S. S. Bush (Eds.), *Mild traumatic brain injury: Symptom Validity Assessment and Malingering* (pp. 231–267). New York, NY: Springer.

Waddell, G. (2004). *The back pain revolution.* Edinburgh, UK: Churchill Livingstone.

Waddell, G., McCulloch, J. A., Kummel, E., & Venner, R. M. (1980). Nonorganic physical signs in low-back pain. *Spine (Phila Pa 1976), 5,* 117–125.

Wang, Y. C., Kapellusch, J., & Garg, A. (2014). Important factors influencing the return to work after stroke. *Work, 47,* 553–559.

Wechsler, D. A. (1997). *Wechsler Adult Intelligence Scale-III.* New York, NY: Psychological Corporation.

Wetter, M. W., & Corrigan, S. K. (1995). Providing information to clients about psychological tests: A survey of attorneys' and law students' attitudes. *Professional Psychology: Research and Practice, 26,* 474–477.

Widows, M. R., & Smith, G. P. (2005). *Structured Inventory of Malingered Symptomatology professional manual.* Odessa, FL: Psychological Assessment Resources.

Williamson, D. J., Holsman, M., Chaytor, N., Miller, J. W., & Drane, D. L. (2012). Abuse, not financial incentive, predicts non-credible cognitive performance in patients with psychogenic non-epileptic seizures. *Clinical Neuropsychologist, 26,* 588–598.

Wilson, R. S., Sytsma, J., Barnes, L. L., & Boyle, P. A. (2016). Anosognosia in dementia. *Current Neurology and Neuroscience Reports, 16,* 77.

Wolfe, F. (2000). For example is not evidence: Fibromyalgia and the law. *Journal of Rheumatology, 27,* 1115–1116.

Wygant, D. B., Anderson, J. L., Sellbom, M., Rapier, J. L., Allgeier, L. M., & Granacher, R. P. (2011). Association of the MMPI-2 restructured form (MMPI-2-RF) validity scales with structured malingering criteria. *Psychological Injury and Law, 4,* 13–23.

Wygant, D. B., Ben-Porath, Y. S., Arbisi, P. A., Berry, D. T. R., Freeman, D. B., & Heilbronner, R. L. (2009). Examination of the MMPI-2 restructured form (MMPI-2-RF) validity scales in civil forensic settings: Findings from simulation and known group samples. *Archives of Clinical Neuropsychology, 24,* 671–680.

Youngjohn, J. R. (1995). Confirmed attorney coaching prior to neuropsychological evaluation. *Assessment, 2,* 279–283.

Youngjohn, J. R., Wershba, R., Stevenson, M., Sturgeon, J., & Thomas, M. L. (2011). Independent validation of the MMPI-2-RF Somatic/Cognitive and Validity scales in TBI litigants tested for effort. *Clinical Neuropsychologist, 25,* 463–476.

Index

AACN (American Academy of Clinical Neuropsychology), 8, 9, 42–43, 71
Abrahams, J. P., 27
ABRP (American Board of Rehabilitation Psychology), 56
AD (Alzheimer's disease), 72–73, 75, 78
Adjustment Validity (K-r) scale, 34
Adnet Bonte, C., 50–51
adverse reaction to feedback, 116–18
advocacy, patient, 90, 92, 98–99
Al-Ashkar, F., 6
Allen, L. M., 3rd, 79
Allen, R. A., 73–74
Alzheimer's disease (AD), 72–73, 75, 78
American Academy of Clinical Neuropsychology (AACN), 8, 9, 42–43, 71
American Board of Rehabilitation Psychology (ABRP), 56
American Educational Research Association, 2
Amlani, A., 112–13
Amsterdam Short-Term Memory Test (ASTMT), 49–50
Anderson, A. M., 76
angry reactions to feedback, managing, 113
APA (2010) Ethics Code, 126–27
APA Handbook of Rehabilitation Psychology, 3–4
Armistead-Jehle, P., 36–37, 76–77, 93

Ashaye, K., 76–77
Ashendorf, L., 35–36
ASTMT (Amsterdam Short-Term Memory Test), 49–50
Ayres, W., 72

Baade, L. E., 44
Bachman, D. L., 77–78
Back-Madruga, C., 35–36, 37
Baker, D. A., 107–8
Baker, W. J., 75
Barker, M. D., 77–78
Bass, C., 109–10, 113
Battery for Health Improvement-2 (BHI-2), 37
Bayard, S., 50–51
BBHI-2 (Brief Battery for Health Improvement-2), 37
Beglinger, L. J., 52–53
Behavioral Assessment Scale for Children-2, 81
behavioral observations, 83
  ethical considerations, 129–30
  overview, 14–15
  in performance validity assessment, 25–26
  in symptom validity assessment, 39
Behavior Rating Inventory of Executive Functioning-Second Edition (BRIEF-2), 81
Behrouz, R., 47

Benbadis, S. R., 47
Bender, H. A., 48, 79–80
beneficence, 128
Ben-Porath, Y. S., 33
Bertakis, K. D., 96
BHI-2 (Battery for Health Improvement-2), 37
Bianchini, K. J., 44, 46–47, 57–59
Bieu, R. K., 36–37
Binder, L. M., 50–51, 60–61
Biondolillo, A., 27–28, 44–45
Bisson, J. I., 111
Blaha, R. Z., 99
Blaskewitz, N., 25, 79–80
Bleijenberg, G., 49–50, 60–61
Boone, K. B., 22–23, 35–36, 37, 46–47
Braddom's Physical Medicine and Rehabilitation, 3–4, 6–7
brain injury/disease
  epilepsy, 47–48
  Huntington disease, 52–53
  multiple sclerosis, 49–52
  overview, 42
  stroke, 45–47
  traumatic brain injury, 17, 24–25, 43–44
Brennan, A., 44, 46–47
Brey, R. L., 61
BRIEF-2 (Behavior Rating Inventory of Executive Functioning-Second Edition), 81
Brief Battery for Health Improvement-2 (BBHI-2), 37
brief instruments, symptom validity scales in, 37–38
Brief Visuospatial Memory Test-Revised (BVMT-R), 24
Brooks, B. L., 46, 48, 72, 80
Brooks, L., 60
Brown, R. S., 55, 122
b Test, 22–23, 46–47
Burton, R. L., 78–79
Bush, S. S., 3–4, 5, 39–40, 42–43, 56, 73–74, 104–5, 135–36
BVMT-R (Brief Visuospatial Memory Test-Revised), 24

California Verbal Learning Test (CVLT), 37
Calloway, J., 78–79
CARB (Computerized Assessment of Response Bias), 37, 60, 62
Carlson, C., 48, 79–80
Carone, D. A., 27–28, 44–45, 48, 72, 89–90, 92, 104–5
case conference, interdisciplinary, 87

case discussions, 86–87, 90–93
case studies
  adverse reaction to feedback, 116–18
  genuine neurological impairment, feedback in case of, 118
  positive reaction to feedback, 114–15
  psychological disorder assessment, 68
CFS (chronic fatigue syndrome), 49–50, 59–60
Chafetz, M. D., 27–28, 44–45, 112–13
ChAMP (Child and Adolescent Memory Profile), 80
Chaytor, N., 102
cheating, 3
Chelune, G., 51
Child and Adolescent Memory Profile (ChAMP), 80
Child Protective Agency (CPA), 112–13
children. *See* pediatric validity assessments
chronic fatigue syndrome (CFS), 49–50, 59–60
chronic nonmalignant pain, 57
clinical interviews, accuracy of patient responses during, 5
coaching, 87–89
cogniform disorder, 65, 102
cogniphobia, 67
cognitive complaints, 16–17
cognitive functioning, 55
cognitive screening measures, 77–78
Coin-in-the-Hand Test, 77
communication, interdisciplinary. *See* interdisciplinary communication
compensation seeking, 7–8
  neurological symptoms and pain, 121–22
  overview, 120
  roles and relationships, 124–26
  validity assessment in forensic contexts, 123–24
competence, 133–35
comprehensive tests of psychopathology and personality, 32–34
Computerized Assessment of Response Bias (CARB), 37, 60, 62
confrontation of malingering patients, 108–9
Connery, A. K., 107–8
Constant, E. L., 60–61
Constantinou, M., 35–36, 79–80
construct validity, 2
content-based invalid responding, 33
content validity, 2
controlled substances, malingering for, 92–93
conversion disorder, 65
Corrigan, S. K., 87–88

Courtney, J. C., 79
CPA (Child Protective Agency), 112–13
criterion validity, 2
criticizing other healthcare providers, 94–95
Crouch, J. A., 44
Cutter, G. R., 49
CVLT (California Verbal Learning Test), 37

Dandachi-FitzGerald, B., 72–73
Dean, A. C., 75
Delayed Recognition (DR) subtest, 17–18
Delis, D. C., 65, 102
Demakis, G. J., 37, 123
dementia, 73–74, 75–78, 82–83
Dementia Profile, 75–76
Denney, R. L., 76–77, 78–79
Deright, J., 72
diagnosis threat, 103
didactics, 86–90
dignity-sparing techniques, 109–10
Dinkins, J. P., 79
disengagement, 105–6
Dismuke, C. E., 96
distraction tests, 25–26
Donders, J., 73–74
Dot Counting Test, 22–23
double-bind approach, 112
DR (Delayed Recognition) subtest, 17–18
Dragon, W. R., 33
Drane, D. L., 48–49, 102
Duff, K., 52–53, 75, 78
Dufrene, M., 112–13
Dunham, K. J., 78–79, 134–35
Dux, M., 24

Eastwood, S., 111
EDSS (Expanded Disability Status Scale), 49
education, 86–90
Effort Index (EI), 52–53, 77–79
Effort Scale (ES), 52–53, 77–79
Eichstaedt, K. E., 48
Eisendrath, S. J., 112
embedded performance validity tests, 23–25
  advantages and disadvantages of, 25
  constructing, 24
  defined, 14–15
  empirical cutoffs, 15–16
  performance patterns, comparing, 24–25
  Reliable Digit Span, 23–24, 25
  sensitivity, specificity, and predictive values, 15–16
  for traumatic brain injury, 44

embedded symptom validity tests, 4
empirical cutoffs for PVTs, 15–16
Enright, J., 78–79
epilepsy, 47–48
ES (Effort Scale), 52–53, 77–79
ethical considerations
  4 A's of ethical practice, 135–36
  interpretation of results, 130–31
  multimethod approaches, 129–30
  organization practices, conflicts from, 131–33
  overview, 128
  suboptimal competence, 133–35
Exaggeration Index of the Auditory Verbal Learning Test-Expanded, 60
Expanded Dementia Profile, 76
Expanded Disability Status Scale (EDSS), 49

face-saving techniques, 111–12
face validity, 2
factitious disorder, 101, 111, 112
Fadil, H., 50–51
Fake Bad Scale. See Symptom Validity Scale
false positives, 15–16, 48
fatigue, 57
  chronic fatigue syndrome, 59–60
  fibromyalgia, 59–60
FBS (Symptom Validity Scale), 33–34, 58–59
FCEs (functional capacity evaluations), 26
feedback
  about factitious disorder, 111
  adverse reaction case study, 116–18
  for children, 107–8
  feedback model, 104–7
  genuine neurological impairment case study, 118
  good-news bad-news approach, 106–7, 108
  for malingering, 108–11
  positive reaction case study, 114–15
Fenton, J. J., 96
Ference, T., 60
fibromyalgia, 59–60
Fifteen Item Test (FIT), 22–23, 50–51
Fischer, J. S., 49
Fleming, A., 6–7, 11, 93
forced choice performance validity tests, 17–22. See also specific tests
Ford, W., 62
forensic contexts
  neurological symptoms and pain, 121–22
  overview, 120
  roles and relationships, 124–26
  validity assessment in, 123–24

forgetfulness, 16–17
Franchow, E. I., 51
Franks, P., 96
Freeman, T., 36–37
freestanding performance validity tests. *See also specific tests*
　defined, 14–15
　empirical cutoffs, 15–16
　forced choice paradigm, 17–22
　memory paradigm, 16–17
　non-forced-choice, 22–23
　sensitivity, specificity, and predictive values, 15–16
　for traumatic brain injury, 44
freestanding psychological validity tests, criteria for, 5
freestanding symptom validity tests, 4, 34–36. *See also specific tests*
Frontal Systems Behavioral Scale (FrSBe), 83
functional capacity evaluations (FCEs), 26

General Memory Impairment Profile (GMIP), 76
genuine neurological impairment, feedback in case of, 118
geriatric validity assessments
　cognitive screening measures, 77–78
　Coin-in-the-Hand Test, 77
　dementia evaluations, 73–74, 75–78, 82–83
　Dementia Profile, 75–76
　General Memory Impairment Profile, 76
　importance of, 72–74
　malingered dementia, 72
　Medical Symptom Validity Test, 75–76
　memory impairments, 78
　oppositional attitude towards, 73
　performance validity assessment methods, 74–78
　symptom validity assessment methods, 82–83
　underreporting of symptoms, 74
Gervais, R. O., 36, 37, 60, 62, 123
Gigante, V. "The Chin", 72
Gill, D., 76–77
Gittelman, D. K., 72–73
Glatz, C., 71–72
Glynn, G., 57–58
GMIP (General Memory Impairment Profile), 76
Gola, T., 75
Goldberg, H. E., 35–36, 37
Gonzalez-Toledo, E., 50–51
good-news bad-news approach, 106–7, 108

Gottfried, L. A., 111
Grayson, R. L., 67
Green, P., 26–27, 36, 48, 62, 76–77, 93
Greiffenstein, M. F., 75
Greve, K. W., 44, 46–47, 57–58, 59, 123
Grills, C. E., 36–37
grip strength, 24–25
Gunstad, J., 122

Halligan, P., 109–10, 113
Handel, R. W., 33
Harth, S., 76–77
Hartman, D. E., 5
Hathaway, S. R., 32
HD (Huntington disease), 52–53
headaches, 67
Heilbronner, R. L., 35, 42–43
Heinly, M. T., 44, 46–47
Henry, M., 76–77
Henry-Heilbronner Index (HHI), 34
Herzberg, D. S., 46–47
Hoelzle, J. B., 77–78
Holsman, M., 102
Hook, J. N., 77–78
Hopkins Verbal Learning Test-Revised (HVLT-R), 24
Horner, M. D., 77–78, 96
hospital administration, interfacing with, 95–96
hostile reactions to feedback, managing, 113
Houston, R. J., 44
Howe, L. L., 76
Huet, E., 72
Huntington disease (HD), 52–53
HVLT-R (Hopkins Verbal Learning Test-Revised), 24

iatrogenesis, 103
ignoring conclusions of other healthcare providers, 95
illness anxiety disorder, 65
Immediate Recognition (IR) subtest, 17–18
Incesu, A. I., 6
informed consent process, 104–5
Infrequency (INF) scale, 81
interdisciplinary communication, 106
　case discussions, 90–93
　didactics, 86–90
　future directions, 96–97
　interactions to avoid, 94–95
　interfacing with hospital administration, 95–96

overview, 85–86
research collaboration, 93
interpretation of results, 130–31
interviews, accuracy of patient responses during, 5
invalid presentations, 6. *See also* feedback; malingering
   angry and hostile reactions, managing, 113
   face-saving techniques, 111–12
   factitious disorder, 101
   iatrogenesis and diagnosis threat, 103
   noncredible explanations, avoiding, 104
   overview, 98
   significant physical and/or psychiatric problems, 101–2
   underreporting, 103–4, 113–14
IR (Immediate Recognition) subtest, 17–18
Iverson, G. L., 60, 67, 104–5

Jerant, A. F., 96
Johnson-Greene, D., 60
Jongen, P. H. J., 49–50, 60–61
journal club series, 87

Karantzoulis, S., 48, 78–80
Kathmann, N., 25, 79–80
Kaufman, D. A., 76
Keary, T. A., 21
Kelley, R. E., 50–51
Kimbrell, T., 36–37
kinesiophobia, 67
Kirk, J. W., 99
Kirkwood, M. W., 46, 72, 73–74, 99, 101, 107–8
Klein Twennaar, M., 76–77
Knoll, J., 109
Kohlmaier, J., 27
K-r (Adjustment Validity) scale, 34
Kulas, J. F., 36–37
Kuroski, K., 79
Kurtzke, J. F., 49

Lamberty, G. J., 65–66
Lange, B. J., 93
Lange, R. T., 37–38
Lanting, S., 78–79
Larrabee, G. J., 42–43, 62
LeBourgeois, H., 108–9
Lees-Haley, P. R., 55, 122–23
lifespan considerations, 70. *See also* geriatric validity assessments; pediatric validity assessments
litigation, 6–7. *See also* forensic contexts

Loring, D. W., 75, 76
Love, J. M., 44, 46–47
L-r (Uncommon Virtues) scale, 34
Lu, P., 22–23, 46–47
lupus, 61–62

MacAllister, W. S., 48, 79–80
malingered pain-related disability (MPRD), 57–59
malingering, 3–4, 7
   Alzheimer's disease, 72–73
   chronic pain, 57
   dementia, 72
   face-saving techniques, 112
   feedback for, 107, 108–11
   forensic contexts, 123
   incentives for, 99
   invalid presentations, 99–100
   for medication, 92–93
   by proxy, 100, 112–13
   pure, 99–100
Marquine, M. J., 77–78
Marshall, P. S., 44
Martelli, M. F., 67
Martin, P. K., 32–33, 34–35, 52
Mathias, C. W., 44
Mazur-Mosiewicz, A., 46
Mazzone, P. J., 6
MBTI (mild traumatic brain injury), 7, 43–44
McCaffrey, R. J., 35–36, 79–80
MCI (Memory Complaints Inventory), 34–36, 82
MCI (mild cognitive impairment), 75, 78
McKinley, J. C., 32
MCMI-3 (Millon Clinical Multiaxial Inventory, 3rd Edition), 32–33
Medical Symptom Validity Test (MSVT), 12–13, 17–19
   for cogniphobia, 67
   dementia evaluations, 75–76
   for epilepsy patients, 48
   modifications of test administration, 27–28
   sandbagging baseline evaluations, 71–72
medication, malingering for, 92–93
Mehra, R., 6
Memory Complaints Inventory (MCI), 34–36, 82
memory paradigm, 16–17
Memory Validity Profile (MVP), 80
MEMRY (Multidimensional Everyday Memory Ratings for Youth), 82
Merckelbach, H., 66, 102–3

Index

Merten, T., 25, 66, 76–77, 79–80, 102–3
mild cognitive impairment (MCI), 75, 78
mild traumatic brain injury (MBTI), 7, 43–44
Miller, J. W., 102
Millis, S. R., 42–43, 122
Millon Clinical Multiaxial Inventory, 3rd Edition (MCMI-3), 32–33
Minnesota Multiphasic Personality Inventory (MMPI), 32–34, 35
Minnesota Multiphasic Personality Inventory-2nd Edition (MMPI-2), 4–5, 32–33, 36–37, 46–47, 58–59
Minnesota Multiphasic Personality Inventory-Adolescent (MMPI-A), 81
Mittenberg, W., 123
MMPI-2 Restructured Form (MMPI-2-RF), 32–34, 58–59, 66
MMPI-A Restructured Form (MMPI-A-RF), 81, 82–83
Molinari, V. A., 73–74
monthly journal club series, 87
Morgan, D., 78–79
Morgan, J. E., 39–40, 42–43
Moroni, C., 50–51
motivation of test-takers, 3
MPRD (malingered pain-related disability), 57–59
MS. *See* multiple sclerosis
MSVT. *See* Medical Symptom Validity Test
Multidimensional Everyday Memory Ratings for Youth (MEMRY), 82
multimethod approaches, 17, 40, 129–30
multiple sclerosis (MS), 49–52
  Expanded Disability Status Scale, 49
  Fifteen Item Test, 50–51
  Multiple Sclerosis Functional Composite, 49
  21-Item Test, 50–51
  Victoria Symptom Validity Test, 51
MVP (Memory Validity Profile), 80

Nakhutina, L., 48, 79–80
National Academy of Neuropsychology (NAN), 8, 42–43, 56
Negative Impression (NIM) scale, 81
negative predictive value (NPV), 16
NEO-FFI-3 (Neuroticism Extraversion Openness-Five Factor Inventory), 83
Neurobehavioral Symptom Inventory (NSI), 37–38
neurological symptoms and pain, 121–22
neuropsychology, validity assessment in, 8
Neuroticism Extraversion Openness-Five Factor Inventory (NEO-FFI-3), 83

Nibbio, A., 50–51
NIM (Negative Impression) scale, 81
non-content-based invalid responding, 33
noncredible explanations, avoiding, 104
non-forced-choice freestanding PVTs, 17, 22–23
nonmaleficence, 128
Non-Verbal MSVT (NV-MSVT), 75–77
Novitski, J., 78–79
NPV (negative predictive value), 16
NSI (Neurobehavioral Symptom Inventory), 37–38
NV-MSVT (Non-Verbal MSVT), 75–77

occupational therapy (OT), 6–7, 11, 93
O'Connell, M. E., 78–79
Odland, A. P., 52
older patients. *See* geriatric validity assessments
O'Mara, H., 108–9
one-on-one meetings, 87
open-forum case discussions, 86–87
ophthalmological examinations, 6
organization practices, ethical conflicts from, 131–33
orthopedic injuries, 62
osteoarthritis, 61
OT (occupational therapy), 6–7, 11, 93
The Oxford Handbook of Rehabilitation Psychology, 3–4

PAI (Personality Assessment Inventory), 32–33
PAI-A (Personality Assessment Inventory-Adolescent), 81, 82
pain disorders
  malingered pain-related disability, 57–59
  neurological symptoms and, 121–22
  rheumatic diseases, 61–62
  validity assessment of, 57–59
Panenka, W., 67
Pankratz, L., 4, 111–12
paradigms
  performance validity tests, 16–17
  symptom validity tests, 31–32
patient advocacy, 90, 92, 98–99
patient satisfaction, 95–96
Paulsen, J. S., 52–53
PDRT (Portland Digit Recognition Test), 59
pediatric validity assessments
  Child and Adolescent Memory Profile, 80
  feedback for, 107–8
  importance of, 71–72
  malingering, 71
  malingering by proxy, 100, 112–13

Memory Validity Profile, 80
modifications of test administration, 79
Multidimensional Everyday Memory Ratings for Youth, 82
performance validity assessment, 79–80
symptom validity assessment, 81, 82
Test of Memory Malingering, 79–80
underreporting of symptoms, 74
Word Memory Test, 79
peer-reviewed journal articles, 87
performance validity
   lack of information on, 2–3
   need for assessment, 6–7
   professional assessment, 8–12
   in research settings and clinical work, 7–8
   terminology, 4
performance validity tests (PVTs). *See also specific tests*
   ancillary issues, 26
   chronic fatigue syndrome assessments, 60
   chronic pain assessments, 57–59
   dementia evaluations, 73–74
   embedded, 23–25
   fibromyalgia assessments, 60
   forced choice freestanding, 17–22
   geriatric validity assessments, 74–78
   interpretation of results, 28
   modifications of test administration, 27–28
   non-forced-choice freestanding, 22–23
   orthopedic and spinal cord injury assessment, 62
   overview, 14
   paradigms, 16–17
   pediatric validity assessments, 72, 79–80
   posttraumatic stress disorder assessments, 37
   psychological disorder assessment, 35
   qualitative assessment of performance validity, 25–26
   rheumatic disease assessments, 61–62
   sensitivity, specificity, and predictive values, 15–16
   terminology, 4–5, 14–15
   traumatic brain injury, 43–44
permission for use of tests, 12–13
personality, comprehensive tests of, 32–34
Personality Assessment Inventory (PAI), 32–33
Personality Assessment Inventory-Adolescent (PAI-A), 81, 82
Peterson, R. L., 107–8
physical problems, invalid presentation of, 101–2
physical therapy (PT), 93
PIM (Positive Impression) scale, 82

Ploetz, D. M., 46, 48
PNES (psychogenic nonepileptic seizures), 48–49, 102
Ponds, R. W., 72–73
Portland Digit Recognition Test (PDRT), 59
positive classifications, false, 15–16
Positive Impression (PIM) scale, 82
positive predictive value (PPV), 16
positive reaction to feedback, 114–15
postconcussion syndrome, 122
posttraumatic stress disorder (PTSD), 36–37, 123
Powell, M., 36–37
PPV (positive predictive value), 16
predictive validity, 2, 15–16
premorbid functioning, 123–24
Prins, J. B., 49–50, 60–61
profession-specific validity tests, 12–13
profile analysis, 44–45, 76, 80–81
psychiatric problems, invalid presentation of, 101–2
psychogenic nonepileptic seizures (PNES), 48–49, 102
psychogenic pseudostroke, 47
psychological disorders, 62–64
   assessment validity, 2
   case illustration, 68
   cogniphobia, 67
   somatic symptoms and related disorders, 65–66
psychopathology, comprehensive tests of, 32–34
psychotic disorders, 36
PT (physical therapy), 93
PTSD (posttraumatic stress disorder), 36–37, 123
pulmonary embolisms, misdiagnosis of, 6
pure malingering, 99–100
Putnam, S. H., 122
PVTs. *See* performance validity tests

qualitative assessment
   in geriatric and pediatric patients, 83
   performance validity tests, 25–26
   symptom validity assessment, 39
quantitative assessment, 56

Randolph, C., 78–79
rapport, building, 104–5
Razani, J., 22–23
RBANS (Repeatable Battery for the Assessment of Neuropsychological Status), 27, 52–53, 77–78
RBS (Response Bias Scale), 33–34
RDS. *See* Reliable Digit Span

rehabilitation psychologists, assessments performed by, 9, 12
Reich, P., 111
Reid, W. H., 72
Reingold, S. C., 49
Reliable Digit Span (RDS), 23–24, 25
　for chronic pain assessment, 59
　dementia evaluations, 75
　for stroke patients, 46
　for traumatic brain injury, 44
Repeatable Battery for the Assessment of Neuropsychological Status (RBANS), 27, 52–53, 77–78
requests to not use validity tests, 94
research collaboration, 93, 96–97
Resnick, P. J., 99–100, 109
respectful confrontation, 109
Response Bias Scale (RBS), 33–34
response validity, 5, 31
rheumatic diseases, 61–62
Rienstra, A., 73–74, 76–77
Rohling, M. L., 37, 62, 123
Roor, J. J., 72–73
Roth, R. S., 86
Rubenzer, S., 36–37
Rucas, K., 6–7, 11, 93
Rudick, R. A., 49
Rush, B. K., 3–4, 5, 56

Sachs, B. C., 76
Salazar, X., 22–23
sandbagging baseline evaluations, 71–72
Sawyer, R. J., 2nd, 24
Schatz, P., 71–72
schizophrenia, 102
Schmand, B., 76–77
Schnellbacher, S., 108–9
Schroeder, R. W., 44, 46, 52
self-report scales, 4–5
Sellbom, M., 66
sensitivity, 15–16
Severe Impairment Profile (SIP), 44–45, 75–76
SGFP (Specialty Guidelines for Forensic Psychology), 126–27
Shadia, S., 78–79
Shafi, R., 11
Shankar, K., 76–77
Sherman, E. M., 46, 80
Sieck, B. C., 52–53
Silverberg, N. D., 67, 77–78
SIMS (Structured Interview of Malingered Symptomatology), 34–35, 36–37

Singhal, A., 76–77
SIP (Severe Impairment Profile), 44–45, 75–76
SIRS (Structured Interview of Reported Symptoms), 36–37
SLE (systemic lupus erythematosus), 61–62
Smith, M. M., 52–53
Sofkoa, C. A., 78–79
somatic symptom disorder, 65–66, 102
Specialty Guidelines for Forensic Psychology (SGFP), 126–27
specificity, 15–16
speeded peg placement, 24–25
Spencer, R. J., 86
Spickard, B., 60–61, 67
spinal cord injuries, 62
Standards for Educational and Psychological Testing, 3
Steele, S., 78–79
stroke, 45–47
　b Test for, 46–47
　Minnesota Multiphasic Personality Inventory-2nd Edition, 46–47
　psychogenic pseudostroke, 47
　Reliable Digit Span, 46
　Test of Memory Malingering, 46
Structured Interview of Malingered Symptomatology (SIMS), 34–35, 36–37
Structured Interview of Reported Symptoms (SIRS), 36–37
Stutts, J. T., 108
Suchy, Y., 51
Suhr, J., 60–61, 67
Suhr, J. A., 122
supportive confrontation, 109–10, 111
SVA. *See* symptom validity assessment
SVTs. *See* symptom validity tests
Sweet, J. J., 42–43
symptom exaggeration, 7
symptom retraining, 111–12
symptom validity
　lack of information on, 2–3
　need for assessment, 6–7
　professional assessment, 8–12
　in research settings and clinical work, 7–8
　terminology, 4
symptom validity assessment (SVA). *See also specific tests*
　freestanding SVTs, 34–35
　fundamental truths about, 39–40
　geriatric validity assessments, 82–83
　overview, 30
　pediatric validity assessments, 72, 79–83

qualitative assessment, 39
SVT paradigms, 31–32
symptom validity scales, 32–34
symptom validity scales, in brief instruments, 37–38
terminology, 31
Symptom Validity Scale (FBS), 33–34, 58–59
symptom validity scales, 32–34
  Brief Battery for Health Improvement-2, 37
  in brief instruments, 37–38
  comprehensive tests of psychopathology and personality, 32–34
  Minnesota Multiphasic Personality Inventory, 32–34
  Neurobehavioral Symptom Inventory, 37–38
symptom validity tests (SVTs). *See also specific tests*; symptom validity scales
  for chronic pain, 58–59
  defined, 31
  embedded, 4
  freestanding, 4, 34–36
  paradigms, 31–32
  posttraumatic stress disorder assessments, 37
  terminology, 4
systemic lupus erythematosus (SLE), 61–62

TBI (traumatic brain injury), 17, 24–25, 43–44
Testa, S. M., 24
Test of Memory Malingering (TOMM), 20
  chronic fatigue syndrome assessments, 60–61
  chronic pain assessments, 59
  dementia evaluations, 75
  epilepsy assessments, 48
  fibromyalgia assessments, 60
  Huntington disease assessments, 53
  orthopedic and spinal cord injury assessments, 62
  pediatric validity assessments, 79–80
  posttraumatic stress disorder assessments, 37
  psychological disorder assessments, 35–36
  stroke assessments, 46
test-taker motivation, 3
test validity, 2, 5
Thorgusen, S. R., 51
Todd, D. D., 67
Tolin, D. F., 36–37
TOMM. *See* Test of Memory Malingering
Trauma Symptom Inventory (TSI), 36–37
traumatic brain injury (TBI), 17, 24–25, 43–44
True Response Inconsistency (TRIN-r) scale, 33

TSI (Trauma Symptom Inventory), 36–37
Turner, T. H., 96
21-Item Test, 50–51
Twumasi-Ankrah, P., 44

Uncommon Virtues (L-r) scale, 34
underreporting, 74, 82, 83, 103–4, 113–14

validity, defining, 2
validity assessment
  in forensic contexts, 123–24
  importance of, 6
  in neuropsychology, 8
  in other professions, 6–7
van der Meer, J. W., 49–50, 60–61
van der Werf, S. P., 49–50, 60–61
VanKirk, K. K., 96
Variable Response Inconsistency (VRIN-r) scale, 33
Victoria Symptom Validity Test (VSVT), 21, 48, 51

Waddell signs, 25–26
Warner-Chacon, K., 22–23
WC (Word Choice) subtest, 22
Wetter, M. W., 87–88
Wetter, S. R., 65, 102
Williamson, D. J., 102
Wilson, P., 99
WMT. *See* Word Memory Test
Wolf, S. A., 76–77
Wolfe, F., 125
Word Choice (WC) subtest, 22
Word Memory Test (WMT), 12–13, 17–18, 26–27
  chronic fatigue syndrome assessments, 60–61
  cogniphobia assessments, 67
  dementia evaluations, 75–77
  epilepsy assessments, 48
  fibromyalgia assessments, 60
  Memory Complaints Inventory scales, comparing to, 35–36
  modifications of test administration, 27–28
  orthopedic and spinal cord injury assessments, 62
  pediatric validity assessments, 79
  posttraumatic stress disorder assessments, 37
Wygant, D. B., 58–59, 66

Youngjohn, J. R., 87–88